Neuroplasticity Made Easy

Jon Adams

Copyright © 2024 Jonathan Adams

All rights reserved.

ISBN: 9798327703926

CONTENTS

1 The Basics of Neuroplasticity .... Pg 6

2 The History and Evolution of Neuroplasticity .... Pg 13

3 Brain Rewiring in Action .... Pg 22

4 Stimulating the Plastic Brain .... Pg 31

5 Neuroplasticitys Dark Side .... Pg 42

6 Technological Advances and Neuroplasticity .... Pg 50

7 Cognitive and Emotional Aspects .... Pg 66

8 The Aging Brain and Plasticity .... Pg 73

9 Future Frontiers in Neuroplasticity .... Pg 83

INTRODUCTION

Welcome to "Neordplasticity Made Easy," your guide to understanding one of the most groundbreaking concepts in brain science. The human brain, once considered a rather static organ, is in truth a dynamic landscape continually reshaped by every thought, experience, and memory—a phenomenon known as neuroplasticity.

Within these pages, we'll unravel the complexities of neuroplasticity, turning intricate scientific knowledge into accessible, actionable insights. You'll embark on a journey through the mind's incredible ability to reorganize pathways, create new connections, and even grow new neurons—a journey relevant to everyone from the curious layman to the seasoned academic.

As we peel back the layers of this fascinating topic, we'll explore not just the theoretical underpinnings but also the practical applications that can benefit your daily life. From enhancing learning and memory to aiding recovery from neurological injuries, neuroplasticity holds immense promise for personal growth and well-being.

Expect to uncover strategies that can harness your brain's plastic nature, whether you're looking to pick up a new skill, improve mental performance, or simply gain a deeper appreciation for the awe-inspiring adaptability of your own cognitive machinery.

Through relatable examples, engaging explanations, and a touch of humor, "Neuroplasticity Made Easy" will equip you with the tools to actively shape your brain's development. Prepare to be enlightened and empowered by the untapped potential residing within your own skull.

THE BASICS OF NEUROPLASTICITY

Neuroplasticity is the brain's natural ability to form and adjust synaptic connections in response to learning and experience. This adaptive process is critical for memory formation, skill acquisition, and recovery from neurological damage. Neuroplasticity enables the brain to compensate for lost function by reorganizing itself, making it a fundamental aspect of brain development and lifelong learning. Its influence extends to various cognitive functions and emotional health, underscoring its importance in our everyday lives. Understanding neuroplasticity allows us to appreciate the brain's capacity for change and can inform strategies to enhance our cognitive well-being.

Neuroplasticity, the brain's capacity for change, plays an integral role in how we learn, adapt, and recover. It allows the brain to modify its connections and rewire itself, not only during childhood but also into adulthood. When we acquire new skills, be it playing a guitar or mastering a new language, our brain changes and adapts. This process involves the strengthening of certain neural pathways that are frequently used and the weakening of those that aren't—much like how a path in a forest becomes clearer with regular use. Healing from brain injuries also hinges on neuroplasticity; the brain compensates for damaged areas by forming new connections, sometimes utilizing different parts of the brain to take over functions. By presenting the science behind neuroplasticity in clear, common-sense language, we uncover a subject deeply rooted in our ability to grow and heal, demonstrating the remarkable adaptability of our most vital organ.

When an individual embarks on learning to play the guitar, their brain initiates a remarkable series of events at a molecular level. Beginning with the strum of a chord, the brain's neurons become active, releasing neurotransmitters like glutamate into the synaptic cleft, the space between neurons. Glutamate binds to receptors on the adjacent neuron, leading to an increase in receptor density, which is crucial for the strengthening of synaptic connections. This activity sets off a cascade of signals that contribute to long-term potentiation (LTP), an enduring increase in signal transmission between neurons.

As LTP unfolds, dendritic spines—tiny protrusions on the surface of neurons—begin to change shape. Some spines retract, and new ones form or stabilize, expanding the neuron's capacity to connect with other neurons. This synaptic remodeling is the physical embodiment of neuroplasticity, where the brain's structure is literally reshaped by experience. Through repetition and practice, these synaptic changes are consolidated; with every repeated melody or riff, the newly formed or fortified pathways become more efficient and reliable.

This biological process underlies the observable improvements in a guitarist's skill set. Enhanced dexterity and muscle memory are behavioral manifestations of the intricate dance of molecules and cells within the brain. As the guitarist becomes more proficient, the brain requires less conscious effort to perform complex finger movements, thanks to the robust neural connections solidified by neuroplasticity. This exemplifies how cellular changes translate into tangible, real-world skills, showcasing the profound capacity of the brain to evolve in response to our actions and experiences.

Imagine the brain as an orchestra, each neuron an accomplished musician ready to contribute to the grand performance of thought, memory, and action. As a musician tunes their instrument, neurons adjust their synaptic connections, fine-tuning their responses through repeated practice and experience. When learning, say, to ride a bike, it's as if a group of string instruments starts to play together, initially finding their rhythm. With practice, their individual notes align, creating a smooth, harmonious tune that reflects a strengthening neural pathway. Just as musicians rehearse to commit a piece to memory, our brain rehearses the motions of pedaling and balancing until the act becomes second nature. It's not about striking a single note but about combining and coordinating many, forming a symphony of connections that lead to the effortless joy of riding without a second thought. This is neuroplasticity in action: a symphony of synapses, creating the beautiful music of our daily lives.

Let's zoom in on what happens in the brain when you're learning to ride a bike, focusing on the tiny yet bustling world of the synapse. Picture each attempt to balance on the bike as a signal sent from one neuron to another, across the synaptic gap—this space is where the magic of learning and memory begins. During this process, glutamate, a key neurotransmitter, is released, like a trumpet blaring its first notes in a rehearsal. Glutamate binds to receptors on the receiving neuron just as a lock clicks open when the right key is inserted.

This binding sparks a series of reactions inside the neuron, not unlike a series of musical scales being practiced. These reactions lead to changes in the strength and efficiency of the synaptic connection, similar to a sound technician optimizing the acoustics for a concert. Long-term potentiation, or LTP, is like the whole orchestra reaching a crescendo—signals are passed along these connections more effectively with each repetition.

As you practice, something else remarkable happens: the insulation around the neurons, called myelin, becomes thicker, the way a musician refines the tone of their instrument. This myelination process ensures the messages travel faster and with greater precision, like a melody line being played with increasing confidence and grace.

Finally, as the pathways in your brain become more established, actions like pushing the pedals and steering the handlebars start to feel automatic. Each time you hop on your bike, the neural symphony plays more harmoniously, leading to that glorious moment when you glide effortlessly down the path, no longer conscious of each individual motion—the concert is a success! This, in a nutshell, is the beauty of neuroplasticity: a composition of synaptic connections that begins with simple notes and evolves into a majestic symphony of mastered skills.

Dr. Michael Merzenich, a remarkable figure who has mapped the ways our brains can adapt and strengthen. Imagine you're visiting a new city with a complex subway system. At first, the map is a tangle of colors and lines. Now, think of your brain like it's learning the routes of this metro. Each day, as you travel, you begin to understand how the lines intersect and where each station is in relation to the city above. This is your brain's incredible ability to form cognitive maps, constantly refining and updating this knowledge as you explore more. Merzenich's research unveils how these mental maps aren't just static pictures but living representations, changing as we learn and remember. By navigating the subway, your brain is strengthening its ability to learn and remember paths – a clear showcase of a neuroplastic brain at work. This process isn't restricted to navigating transit; it's how we learn most things in life, from languages to sports, each one like discovering a new route that gets easier the more we travel it. Through Dr. Merzenich's insights, we see our brain's potential to grow and modify itself with each new experience, keeping us on the right track no matter where we're headed.

Let's unpack the intricacies of Dr. Michael Merzenich's work on neuroplasticity and how it's not so different from mastering the labyrinthine subway on your first visit to a sprawling metropolis. As you familiarize yourself with the subway, your brain is doing something quite extraordinary at a cellular level. Every time you remember a route, your brain cells, or neurons, communicate through tiny structures called synapses. The frequent use of a particular route in the subway helps you remember the way more easily over time—this is synaptic plasticity in action.

In the brain, key players in this process are proteins known as NMDA and AMPA receptors located at the synapse. Think of these receptors as the turnstiles of a subway station, controlling the flow of passengers—in this case, neurotransmitters like glutamate. With constant use, turnstiles (receptors) become more efficient, letting through the right amount of neurotransmitters to strengthen the connection between neurons, like a well-practiced commuter swiftly passing through a station.

This enhanced passing of signals at synapses contributes to a stronger and more accurate cognitive map in the hippocampus, akin to keeping a crisp, detailed map in your pocket, which helps you navigate the city better each day. Over time, the impact of these reinforced synapses is supported by neurotrophic factors—proteins that serve to nourish and maintain neurons, much as a seasoned traveler learns to pack efficiently for smoother journeys.

Neurogenesis, the birth of new neurons, also plays a part, continually adding fresh perspectives to your cognitive map, just as city planners might update subway maps with new lines or stations. This vibrant neuroscientific landscape of learning and adaptation is akin to the constant flux and flow of a city in motion, with each neuron, each synapse, each neural pathway contributing to the intricate, awe-inspiring network of a living, learning brain. Through this lens, we can begin to appreciate the profound complexity and sheer beauty of our own neuroplastic minds—capable of not just memorizing routes but transforming every new experience into a seamless journey of growth.

Consider your brain as a garden you're cultivating. Just as you'd plant seeds in rich soil, initiating new skills starts by introducing the basics to your brain. Each effort you make, every practice session you conduct, is like watering these seeds and ensuring they get enough sunlight to thrive. Over time, these actions, these consistent doses of care, strengthen the neural pathways associated with your new abilities, much in the same way a sapling grows stronger and sturdier. Regularly engaging with your new skill is akin to the diligent gardener tending to their plants, encouraging a bloom of colorful flowers. As you practice and repeat what you've learned, the 'garden' of your brain fills with the 'flora' of knowledge and expertise, displaying the visible fruits of your labor. Remember, both gardens and brains need ongoing nurturing to flourish—there are no shortcuts to a blossoming bed of flowers or mastering a new language or instrument.

Here's the breakdown of what happens in your brain's 'garden' when you're learning something new, like starting a vegetable patch from scratch:

- **Sowing the Seeds (Initial Learning)**
  - Introduce the basics of a new skill, and your brain's neurons start firing in specific patterns, like planting seeds in carefully plotted rows ready for growth.
  - Each initial effort lights up a part of the brain, forming the foundation of a neural pathway, much as a seedling emerges from the soil.

- **Watering and Sunlight (Practice and Reinforcement)**
  - Regular practice of the skill waters these new neural seedlings, helping to establish the pathways.
  - Glial cells act like the garden's ecosystem, supporting neurons by providing them with nutrients and removing waste, keeping neural pathways 'fertile'.
  - The continuous practice triggers a series of reactions leading to stronger synapses – it's the fertilizer strengthening the budding plants.

- **Growth and Strengthening (Synaptic Plasticity)**
  - Like a plant's roots reaching into the earth, neural connections deepen and spread as long-term potentiation (LTP) occurs, bolstering the pathways that we use more often.
  - Dendritic spines grow and form new synapses like offshoots of a maturing plant, increasing the richness of the neural network.

- **Blooming (Mastery and Memory)**
  - The hippocampus, our memory's central garden, consolidates these strengthened pathways into long-term retention, allowing a once complex task to be completed with ease and less conscious thought – much like an experienced gardener intuitively knows the rhythms of their garden.
  - Repetition is key; the more you practice, the more second nature the

skill becomes, just as a blooming garden becomes a tapestry of colors each season with regular maintenance.

- **Ongoing Care (Continuous Maintenance and Learning)**
    - Just as a garden requires ongoing care, continuous learning ensures that the brain's pathways remain healthy and pliable.
    - Neurogenesis keeps the brain growing new neural 'plants', demonstrating that the garden of the mind never stops growing, regardless of age.

Each step in the learning process is dynamic, a testament to the brain's ability to adapt and expand. It's not just about planting an idea and watching it grow; it's about how we tend to our mental garden through practice and persistence, creating a lush landscape of knowledge and skills that stays with us for a lifetime.

The field of neuroplasticity is advancing at an impressive speed, with recent research shedding light on how we might improve the brain's ability to reform and adapt. Brain-machine interfaces (BMIs) stand at the forefront of this frontier. These devices connect directly with brain tissue, picking up electrical signals and translating them into actions, like moving a prosthetic limb just by thinking about it. This works because the devices tap into the brain's existing plasticity, creating a two-way communication system that allows the brain to learn and work with artificial extensions of the body.

Meanwhile, neuroimaging technologies such as fMRI and PET scans are becoming more advanced, providing detailed maps of brain activity that offer insights into neuroplastic changes as they happen. Researchers can now observe which areas of the brain light up during specific tasks, and even see the physical changes that occur during the learning process.

The combination of these tools not only deepens our understanding of the brain's inner workings but opens up exciting possibilities for rehabilitation and enhancement. With these technologies, we can envision a future where learning is accelerated, the damage from injuries is more efficiently repaired, and neurodegenerative diseases are better managed. It's a world where the boundary between human and machine blurs in the service of health and human potential, offering a new realm of possibilities that were once confined to science fiction. As these tools improve, the crucial balance lies in harnessing their power to complement and augment our brain's natural abilities without overwhelming or oversimplifying the complex majesty of the human mind.

Brain-machine interfaces (BMIs) tap into the brain's natural ability to rewire itself, a feature known as neuroplasticity, to translate thoughts into action. Here's how: first, BMIs detect electrical signals emitted by the brain when it is engaged in a task or thought. These signals, generated by neurons firing in specific patterns, are captured by implanted electrodes or external sensors. Sophisticated algorithms analyze the timing and frequency of these signals, decoding them into commands that a computer or prosthetic limb can understand. For instance, when a person with a prosthetic arm imagines moving their hand, the corresponding neural activity is converted into movements of the artificial limb. Through feedback and practice, the brain learns to fine-tune these signals, enhancing the cohesion between thought and prosthetic response – this is neuroplasticity in action.

Parallel to this, neuroimaging tools like functional MRI (fMRI) provide a window into the brain's activity during such tasks by tracking changes in blood flow, essentially mapping which areas become more active and require more oxygen. Similarly, positron emission tomography (PET) scans introduce a low-level radioactive tracer into the bloodstream; as it travels to active brain regions, the tracer emits positrons, which are detected by the scanner. This offers insight into the metabolic activity of brain cells undergoing change during neuroplasticity. Together, these technologies not only augment human capabilities but also deepen our understanding of the remarkable adaptability of our brains.

In conclusion, the concept of neuroplasticity is not just a scientific fact, but a gateway to personal empowerment. It presents an essential truth: through determined effort and targeted training, each individual possesses the capacity to rewire their brain. Whether the goal is to master a new skill, recover from injury, or reimagine your life's path, the plasticity of the brain is the foundation upon which change is built. This understanding ushers in a call to approach our brain's adaptability with a sense of wonder and proactive engagement. Embrace the knowledge that with dedication, the brain's dynamic nature can be directed towards meaningful change, ensuring that the journey of self-improvement and resilience is a continuous and rewarding one.

THE HISTORY AND EVOLUTION OF NEUROPLASTICITY

At the dawn of neuroplasticity, the scientific community's doubts mirrored the skepticism faced by the Wright brothers before their historic flight. Just as the concept of a flying machine was initially dismissed, the notion that the adult brain could flex and mold itself was met with caution and suspicion. Critics then, much like those witnessing the Wright brothers prepare for lift-off, couldn't fathom the possibilities beyond the accepted limits; they clung to the view that the brain's pathways were as fixed as railway tracks. However, just as the Wright brothers' success at Kitty Hawk shattered the belief that human flight was impossible, pioneering experiments gradually lifted neuroplasticity to its rightful place in science. It showcased the brain's latent agility, much like an airplane's graceful maneuvers in the sky—a testament to the power of persistence and the potential for change, both in the skies and within the folds of the human brain.

Here is the detailed breakdown of the formative stages in neuroplasticity's scientific saga:

- **Acceptance and Resistance Stages**
  - **Initial Skepticism and Rejection**
    - The early conception of neuroplasticity was met with significant doubt, similar to the skepticism one might encounter when suggesting smartphones could one day replace personal computers.
  - **Gradual Accumulation of Evidence**
    - As studies trickled in, the evidence began to mound, much like a snowball effect, where each layer adds to a larger, undeniable mass.

- **Key Experiments**
  - **Study Designs**
    - Many studies employed controlled lab environments where animal models were subjected to varying stimuli to observe potential changes in the brain's structure or function, mirroring the way we might test the durability of different materials under stress.

- **Hypotheses and Findings**
  - Hypotheses often centered on proving the brain could change with experience or after injury, and results consistently pointed to this conclusion, echoing the way repeated experiments reinforce a scientific theory.
- **Impact on Neuroscientific Viewpoints**
  - Each successful experiment challenged the prevailing doctrine of a static brain, gradually turning the tide in much the same way a string of successful underdog victories can change the outlook of a sports season.

- **Milestone Accomplishments**
  - **Groundbreaking Studies**
    - Seminal research included studies on brain changes following environmental enrichment in animals or altered sensory input in humans, which can be likened to observing the effects of a specialized training regimen on an athlete's performance.
  - **Publications that Shifted Paradigms**
    - Influential papers and books that synthesized research findings served as pivotal moments, much like landmark legal rulings that redefine the interpretation of laws.
  - **Adoption of Neuroplastic Concepts in Medical Treatments**
    - The acceptance of neuroplastic principles led to new therapeutic approaches for stroke recovery, brain injuries, and learning disorders, akin to the way GPS technology transitioned from military to civilian use, revolutionizing navigation for the general public.

Each piece of this puzzle offered a deeper understanding of the brain's malleability. Standing now on the vantage point of current knowledge, one can look back with appreciation at the journey neuroplasticity has undertaken, from a dismissible hypothesis to a cornerstone of contemporary neuroscience—much like we view the shift from gaslight to the ubiquity of electric light. It's a shining example of the progress born from questioning and surpassing the limits of accepted knowledge.

Santiago Ramón y Cajal stands as a monumental figure in the study of neuroplasticity. His groundbreaking work in the late 19th and early 20th centuries provided the first detailed illustrations and hypotheses about the structure of the nervous system. Cajal proposed that neurons are separate entities, not continuous with one another, defying the prevailing belief of the time. This concept, known as the "neuron doctrine," established that neurons communicate with one another via synapses. His persistence, despite initial resistance, propelled forward the understanding that the brain is not a static organ but can change with experience—a process we now call neuroplasticity.

Cajal meticulously documented his observations through precise drawings, laying a foundation that others would build upon with more modern technologies such as electron microscopy and neuroimaging. By meticulously observing individual neurons, he discovered they grow and form new connections—a premise that was critical for later researchers who showed that the brain can rewire itself after injury or through learning.

Today, Cajal's theories are not only confirmed but form the bedrock upon which fields like neuropsychology and neurorehabilitation rest. It's his spirit of curiosity and determination that inspires current neuroscience, guiding us to explore beyond the seen and known, and appreciate the ever-evolving capability of the human brain.

Let's take a closer look at Santiago Ramón y Cajal's trailblazing research, which was much like navigating a maze with only a candle to light the way. He ingeniously harnessed the Golgi stain technique, which, by selectively darkening a few neurons among the forest of cells, brought into stark relief the intricate pathways neurons formed. Picture a solitary lighthouse beam revealing only certain ships on a vast ocean, each ship representing a neuron. This method allowed him to see that neurons stood apart from each other, rather than forming continuous blends as reticular theory suggested.

Cajal was meticulous, sketching the exposed neurons with such artistry and precision that his drawings are still revered today. Just as a cartographer painstakingly maps uncharted land, Cajal's illustrations provided visual proof of neurons' independence. He outlined the life of neurons—how they reach out with their axons and dendrites, much like branches and roots of a tree, to communicate at points we now know as synapses, where the exchange of information occurs through an elegant chemical dance.

His conclusions were radical for the time, countering the reticular theory, which postulated that the nervous system was a large, physically interconnected network. Instead, Cajal proposed that each neuron is a discrete entity, relaying messages to its neighbors in a tightly controlled and precise manner—revolutionizing our understanding of brain circuitry.

The immediate impact of Cajal's work reverberated throughout neuroscience. It wasn't just that he sketched neurons; he unveiled a network that was much more flexible and individualized than previously imagined. His discoveries paved the way for the concept of neuroplasticity—the idea that these connections among neurons are not fixed, but rather can be rewired in response to learning or injury.

Moreover, Cajal's insights set the stage for electron microscopy, which would later visualize synapses at an even smaller scale, revealing their complexity and confirming his theories. By establishing that the brain's communication system could be remapped, he heralded new approaches in rehabilitation and underscored the potential for the brain to recover and adapt. Cajal's work, thus, laid the first stones on the path to modern neuroscience, a discipline forever in debt to his vision and resolve, a field continually inspired by the principles he deduced over a century ago.

As we delve into the landmark studies that signified a turning point for neuroplasticity, it's much like piecing together a complex puzzle that revealed the double helix structure of DNA—each study providing crucial insight into the brain's capacity to adapt. These studies explored various aspects of neuroplasticity, from neuronal growth after environmental enrichment to the brain's ability to reroute functions post-injury.

One influential study observed how rats raised in stimulating environments developed thicker cortexes compared to those in deprived settings, indicating that the brain's structure could be influenced by external factors. Another pivotal experiment demonstrated that the adult brain could form new neuronal connections, refuting the idea that neurogenesis was solely a youthful process.

Together, these studies forged a new understanding in neuroscience, similar to realizing that DNA was the blueprint of genetics. They showed that our brains are not rigidly predetermined by our genetics but are instead dynamic entities capable of changing and learning throughout our lives. This knowledge has profound implications, influencing everything from educational practices to rehabilitation therapies, emphasizing that the brain is resilient and capable of remapping pathways, a testament to the malleable nature of our most complex organ.

Neuroplasticity research has evolved through a series of methodical steps, each building upon the findings of the last, much like updates to a complex software system. Let's guide you through this progression:

Early animal studies set the stage, investigating the effects of enriched environments—a space replete with toys and stimuli—against deprived ones. Researchers hypothesized that sensory and cognitive stimulation would affect brain structure. They found that rats in enriched environments indeed had thicker cortices and enhanced synaptic density, suggesting that the brain physically adapts to its surroundings.

Attention then shifted to understanding how the brain's wiring changes in response to learning. Experiments often involved training animals to complete new tasks while monitoring changes in their neuronal circuitry. Findings revealed increased synaptic strength and the formation of new connections in regions associated with the learned behavior, reinforcing the idea that practice can physically reshape our brain's networks.

The techniques became finer, with synaptic plasticity assays measuring the changes in neuron-to-neon communication. These studies confirmed that not only can synapses change their strength, but they can also form entirely new connections or even retract existing ones, demonstrating a level of synaptic flexibility previously unimagined.

In brain injury models, scientists observed how one area of the brain could assume the functions of a damaged one, indicative of the brain's ability to reorganize itself post-injury. This was critical in debunking the idea that each brain area is hardwired for a single purpose without the capacity for adaptation.

These foundational studies and methodologies collectively ushered in a new understanding of the brain's dynamic nature. It's now recognized that neurogenesis—the creation of new neurons—occurs throughout life, not just during development. This realization has had transformative implications for developing therapeutic strategies, suggesting that the brain has a lifelong potential to recover from injury and adapt to new challenges.

As we continue to decode the mysteries of the brain, the lessons from neuroplasticity research stand as pivotal milestones, informing how we approach everything from education to recovery from neurological conditions, painting a picture of a brain that is ever-changing, adaptable, and full of potential.

The consensus on neuroplasticity didn't come overnight, much like the gradual acceptance of any revolutionary technology we use today, like smartphones or the internet. At first, the idea that our brains could be malleable throughout our lives existed on the periphery, much like the early days of personal computers when the potential of digital technology was only beginning to be realized. Over time, compelling evidence from laboratories around the world began to stack up, showing that the brain could indeed form new connections and reorganize itself following injury or through learning, much like updates to software that add new features or improve functionality.

This research made its way into mainstream clinical practices, transforming the prophetic vision into a foundational principle, just as email has transitioned from a novel concept to a staple of our daily communication. Neuroplasticity now underpins modern approaches to rehabilitation, where therapies are designed with the understanding that the brain can relearn and recover functions. We see this when stroke survivors regain mobility or when cognitive techniques are employed to manage neurological conditions, mirroring the way GPS transformed navigation, turning once-complex tasks into intuitive, standard practices.

No longer a novelty, neuroplasticity is today a cornerstone of neuroscience, with methods and applications as widespread and integral as wireless internet: once novel, now indispensable. It is a testament to the idea that, with time, even the most groundbreaking concepts can become woven into the fabric of everyday life, enhancing and enriching our interactions with the world and with ourselves.

Here is the breakdown on the history of neuroplasticity, laid out like the chapters of an unfolding story that leads us to a deeper understanding of our own brains:

- **Tracking the Earliest Inquiries into Neuroplasticity**
  - **Initial Hypotheses and Experiments**

- Early twentieth-century investigations suspected that the brain could adapt after injuries, akin to how a city's traffic system reroutes itself when a main bridge is out.

- Detailing Major Contributions and the Researchers Behind Them
- Noteworthy Publications
- Seminal texts include Donald Hebb's "The Organization of Behavior," which introduced the idea that neurons that fire together wire together—like dancers who learn to move in unison with practice.
- Seminal Conferences or Presentations
- Conferences like the Society for Neuroscience Annual Meeting began to feature neuroplasticity, bringing it from the lab bench nearer to the clinic.

- Describing Landmark Studies that Shifted the Paradigm
- Specific Methodologies Used
- Researchers employed techniques like functional magnetic resonance imaging (fMRI) to observe how learning new tasks can physically change the brain's structure, much as a well-worn path forms in a meadow from repeated use.
- Results and Conclusions Drawn
- The results consistently demonstrated the brain's adaptability, challenging the view that adult brains are incapable of significant change, overturning decades of dogmatic beliefs.

- Explaining the Integration of Neuroplasticity into Clinical Practices
- New Therapies Based on Neuroplastic Principles
- Innovative interventions such as constraint-induced movement therapy for stroke recovery have shown that the brain can be coaxed to reassign functions, like repairing an old car with new, adaptive parts.
- Case Studies Showcasing the Efficacy of These Approaches
- Patient recovery stories serve as testimonials to these plastic changes, illustrating the practical applications of neuroplasticity in tangible ways.

The narrative arc of neuroplasticity is one of gradual acceptance and expansion, from ignored and doubted beginnings to critical relevance and implementation. It's akin to watching a slow-motion dawn break over the field of neuroscience, each ray of light bringing clarity to how we perceive and can potentially heal the human brain. With each new discovery, we continue to map out this terra incognita, revealing that our brains—and hence we—have the lifelong capacity to learn, adapt, and recover.

Neuroplasticity today informs numerous aspects of rehabilitation by underlining the brain's ability to adapt and mend. For instance, in stroke recovery, exercises designed to stimulate affected brain regions are commonly used, helping patients regain functions like speech and motor control. It's like rerouting traffic after a roadblock—therapies encourage the brain to find new pathways to restore its capabilities.

Looking ahead, neuroplasticity's principles could reshape education and technology, personalizing learning to match each individual's brain changes as they acquire new information. Imagine a classroom where educational tools are tailored not just to the topics students need to learn, but also to the ways their brains best process and retain information, much like a fitness regimen customized to one's physiological response.

Moreover, advancements in technology might one day allow us to enhance learning and memory through non-invasive brain stimulation, fine-tuning the brain's circuitry like a technician refining a complex machine. In all these applications, neuroplasticity offers a roadmap to not just recovery but also enhancement, promising a future where learning is more efficient and recovery more complete.

Let's take a deeper look at the rehabilitation therapies guided by the principles of neuroplasticity. Constraint-induced movement therapy (CIMT), for example, involves restricting the use of the unaffected limb, which encourages patients to use the affected side, thereby promoting neural reorganization and functional improvement akin to a person learning to write with their non-dominant hand. Studies have shown significant recovery of motor skills in stroke survivors who engage in this type of training.

Mirror therapy, on the other hand, uses a reflective surface to create the illusion that the affected limb is moving normally. This visual cue can stimulate the brain to "rethink" the motor pathways that were damaged, much like using a GPS to find a new route when the usual one is blocked.

In education, the principles of neuroplasticity are inspiring the creation of adaptive learning technologies, smart programs that alter their teaching strategies based on a learner's performance, not unlike a personal tutor who tailors their instruction methods to a student's unique way of understanding.

Looking at the frontier of cognitive enhancement, techniques like transcranial magnetic stimulation (TMS) show tremendous promise. TMS non-invasively directs magnetic energy to specific brain regions, potentially strengthening or weakening synaptic connections to enhance cognitive abilities, in the same way that exercising a muscle group can improve its strength and function.

The potential of these neuroplasticity-informed therapies and technologies is vast, offering hope for recovery and enhancement that was once unimaginable. The evidence for their effectiveness continues to grow, painting a future where the human brain's adaptability is not only understood but harnessed for remarkable transformation.

Paul Bach-y-Rita was a pioneering figure who translated the concept of neuroplasticity into tangible rehabilitation tools. Through his invention, the BrainPort device, individuals with visual impairments could perceive visual information through tactile sensations on their tongues. His work demonstrated the brain's remarkable ability to interpret sensory data in new ways, exemplifying the plasticity of neural pathways.

Edward Taub's contributions to neuroplasticity are equally significant. His development of constraint-induced movement therapy for patients with paralysis has redefined rehabilitation. By using the unaffected limb less and engaging the affected limb more, he showed that the brain could rewire itself to regain lost functions, providing hope for recovery to countless individuals who had experienced debilitating strokes and injuries.

Understanding neuroplasticity is not just an academic pursuit; it is a revelation about our own potential. The brain's ability to adapt, to form new connections, and even to reassign functions is a powerful testament to our innate capacity for change. As you reflect on this, recognize that each new skill learned, each habit changed, and each recovery from setback, however small, is a demonstration of this incredible cerebral flexibility. Let this knowledge be a source of motivation to continually learn, grow, and embrace life's challenges, knowing that with effort and time, the brain can and will adapt.

BRAIN REWIRING IN ACTION

When our brain's rewire, the ability is not confined to abstract theory but is vividly demonstrated through personal triumphs and the subtle, yet profound, daily advances in learning. We will explore the mechanisms behind this remarkable capacity, revealing how the brain's ability to adapt not only plays a crucial role in recovery from injury but also in the continuous process of acquiring knowledge and skills. From striking tales of healing to the incremental growth of everyday experiences, these narratives showcase neuroplasticity's profound effect on human lives, offering insights into the brain's potential for transformation and the hope it holds for the future.

Neuroplasticity is the brain's ability to reorganize itself by forming new neural connections throughout life. This flexibility enables the brain to adjust to new situations, learn from experiences, and recover from injuries. When one learns a new skill, such as playing the piano, the repeated activity stimulates specific neural pathways, which strengthens them over regular practice. Similarly, after an injury like a stroke, undamaged parts of the brain can sometimes take over the functions that the harmed areas previously managed. It's a continuous and dynamic process that occurs at various levels, from cellular changes, like the growth of new neurons, to large-scale cortical remapping, which can result in shifts in functional areas of the brain. Understanding neuroplasticity is crucial as it underpins many therapeutic approaches for brain injuries and is a cornerstone of ongoing research into improving learning and memory throughout life.

Let's take a deeper look at neuroplasticity by zooming in on what happens at the microscopic level in our brains. Imagine a bustling city where new buildings are constantly constructed (neurogenesis), connections between these buildings are formed (synaptogenesis), and occasionally, underused buildings are taken down to make space for more useful ones (synaptic pruning).

During neurogenesis, the brain forms new neurons, a process once thought to be confined to our early years but now known to occur throughout our lives. Synaptogenesis then takes over, creating connections between neurons, much like building roads or bridges between new structures in a city. The strength of these connections is not static—they are reinforced with frequent use, similar to paths that become more prominent and well-trodden the more they're walked on. This is the essence of synaptic plasticity; synapses can grow stronger or weaker based on how much they are used.

Molecular signals involved in these processes are like the messages sent between construction workers and architects, guiding the development and maintenance of the brain's structure. Brain-derived neurotrophic factor (BDNF), for instance, is akin to a delivery of building materials that promotes the growth of new neurons and strengthens their connections.

Various lifestyle factors, such as environmental enrichment—analogous to having a rich, stimulating city environment, physical exercise—like doing regular construction work to improve city infrastructure, and cognitive challenges—similar to solving complex puzzles to keep the city running efficiently, can all enhance neuroplasticity.

To track these changes, scientists use technologies akin to high-tech tools in urban planning. Functional magnetic resonance imaging (fMRI) lets researchers monitor the brain's activity in real-time, observing which neural pathways light up during different tasks. Neuron tracing techniques are like GPS for the brain, allowing scientists to map out precisely how different regions are interconnected.

Through understanding the fine details of neuroplasticity, we glimpse the incredible adaptability and resilience of our brains, capable of learning and recovering throughout our lives. This knowledge empowers us, offering hope for rehabilitation and the potential for enhancing our cognitive abilities beyond what we ever thought possible.

Imagine your brain as a dynamic metropolis, bustling with traffic, where new routes can be established and old ones improved with each new experience—a city that never stops evolving. This is the very essence of neuroplasticity that Paul Bach-y-Rita tapped into when he helped people with visual impairments 'see' using their tongues. It's as if he found a detour for the visual information, rerouting it through a different sensorial pathway, proving that when one route is blocked, the brain can find another way.

Edward Taub's work with constraint-induced movement therapy (CIMT) further illustrates neuroplasticity's real-world impact. By restricting the use of a patient's unaffected limb, much like closing off a main road to force traffic through smaller streets, he compelled the brain to strengthen neural pathways that controlled the affected limb. This therapy showcases the brain's ability to adapt and retrain itself, much like a person learning to navigate a new city learns the streets by exploring them.

Both these icons of neuroplasticity embody the principle that our brains are not rigidly mapped but are fluid, like a sophisticated network that's continuously updated and optimized, responding to the challenges and demands of our actions and environments.

Here's the lowdown on the profound neurological changes brewing beneath the surface during sensory substitution and constraint-induced movement therapy, all thanks to the brain's neuroplasticity:

- **Sensory Substitution:**
  - **The redirection of sensory input**:
    - Picture the brain as a command center in an emergency situation, swiftly rerouting incoming information to unoccupied operators. This is akin to how sensory substitution works, diverting, for instance, visual data to tactile processing units, allowing a different sense to take over a lost function.
  - **Development of neural pathways for processing alternative sensory information**:
    - Just as a small footpath can widen into a highway with increased use, these alternative sensory pathways can strengthen and become more efficient the more they are used, enabling the brain to perform remarkable feats like 'seeing' through touch.
  - **The role of neuroplasticity in sensory remapping**:
    - Neuroplasticity allows this sensory re-routing to be possible, much like how a city's infrastructure adapts over time, constructing new routes and demolishing unused ones to support changing traffic patterns.

- **Constraint-Induced Movement Therapy (CIMT):**
  - **The principle of 'use it or lose it' in neuroplasticity**:
    - Think of your brain as a member of a sports team; if not given playtime, skills can fade. In CIMT, the unaffected limb is sidelined, encouraging the brain to focus on the affected limb, thereby strengthening

its game.
- **Strategies for promoting use of the affected limb**:
- This is comparable to forcing a left-handed person to use only their right hand, which can be challenging initially, but eventually leads to improvement in right-hand dexterity.
- **Neurological outcomes of CIMT, such as increased cortical representation of the limb**:
- As with muscles that grow with resistance training, the cognitive focus on the affected limb leads to an increase in its representation and function within the brain's 'muscle', the cerebral cortex.

Both therapeutic approaches capitalize on the brain's capacity for change, encouraging the formation and reinforcement of new neurological pathways. At the synaptic level, this involves increasing the number and strength of synaptic connections, similar to upgrading the bandwidth of your internet connection; the more you use it, the better it gets. As a result, the brain's network becomes more robust and intricate, fine-tuned to accommodate new ways of interpreting the world, showcasing the brain's remarkable ability to not just heal and adapt but to essentially reinvent itself.

Consider your daily routine: each task, from preparing a meal to solving a puzzle, is like a puzzle piece in the vast jigsaw of your brain's development. Every time you cook a new recipe, it's like adding a new tool to your culinary toolbox; similarly, your brain forms and strengthens pathways needed for this activity. When you navigate a new route to work, it's not just your car or feet taking a different path, your brain cells blaze a trail too. These activities, as mundane as they might seem, are the brain's workout sessions—flexing its synaptic connections, building mental muscles, and enhancing cognitive maps. Just as a musician practices scales to perfect their craft, so too does your brain refine its abilities through repeated, varied activities, continuously rewiring and developing with each new experience and challenge.

Here's the rundown on the fascinating neural ballet that unfolds in your head when you engage in tasks that are as everyday as making your morning coffee:

- **Cooking a New Recipe:**
- **Engagement of sensory perception and memory recall:**
- Think of each ingredient as a unique note in a symphony. Your brain orchestrates the smell, taste, and texture, retrieving memories of flavors to create a harmonious dish.

- **Integration of fine motor skills and spatial reasoning:**
    - Just as a dancer practices complex moves, your hands and fingers must coordinate precisely, spatially arranging ingredients and utensils, refining your dexterity and coordination each time you cook.
- **Strengthening of neural pathways related to executive function and multitasking:**
    - Managing a kitchen requires planning and multitasking, like a skilled conductor leading a chaotic orchestra to produce a melodious concert, shaping your brain's executive functions to manage complex tasks effortlessly.

- **Navigating a New Route:**
    - **Activation of the hippocampus for spatial navigation and memory:**
    - As a captain relies on their mental map to navigate the seas, your hippocampus charts the course, laying down cognitive maps of new landscapes and the routes through them.
    - **Adaptability and problem-solving processes in the prefrontal cortex:**
    - Finding your way through unexpected detours is a puzzle your brain loves to solve, akin to a detective piecing together clues. Each successful navigation sharpens this problem-solving prowess.
    - **Enhancement of the brain's cognitive 'map' with new geospatial information:**
    - Every new byway and landmark added to your internal GPS enriches your brain's geographical database, akin to updates downloaded to your navigation app, making future journeys smoother and more instinctive.

Diving into the world of neurochemicals, the release of neurotransmitters like dopamine plays the role of a cheering crowd, reinforcing the joy of successful tasks. Each rush of dopamine during these activities not only marks a satisfying achievement but also boosts motivation, encouraging you to repeat, refine, and thus strengthen those neural connections further. It's the brain's own system of positive reinforcement, ensuring that the more you practice a skill, the more proficient you become – a truly elegant system designed for endless learning and adaptation.

Meet John, whose story unfolds like a phoenix rising from ashes, a testament to the brain's incredible capacity for recovery. After a severe stroke, John faced a future where the simple acts of moving his right arm or speaking clear sentences seemed as distant as mountains on the horizon. Through intensive, neuroplasticity-driven therapy, akin to a relentless blacksmith hammering away to reshape and restore a once-dulled blade, John began the slow process of reawakening dormant neural pathways and forging new ones.

Months of dedicated rehabilitation, akin to a gardener diligently tending to a once-wilted plant, brought signs of life back to his limbs. Words that once stumbled on his tongue began to flow more easily, mirroring the way a stream carves its path through the landscape, gradually but powerfully. John's improvement wasn't merely a stroke of luck; it was the direct result of harnessing his brain's malleability—proof that with time, patience, and the right therapeutic approach, even brains that have suffered significant injuries can find a way to heal and regain lost functions.

Stories like John's are lanterns in the dark, illuminating the path for countless others touched by brain injury, showing that the journey back to oneself, while unique for each, is rooted in the shared soil of neuroplasticity.

Here is the breakdown on the intricate therapies and behind-the-scenes neurological changes that fuel the remarkable process of stroke recovery:

- **Types of Neuroplasticity Therapies:**
  - **Constraint-Induced Movement Therapy**:
    - Imagine your unaffected arm is tied down, like a runner with one shoe. This forces you to use the affected arm, gradually improving its dexterity and function.
  - **Motor Imagery**:
    - The patient mentally rehearses a physical movement, similar to an athlete visualizing a perfect run before the race starts, to 'wake up' the brain areas responsible for the actual movement.
  - **Repetitive Task-Specific Training**:
    - Through repeated performance of daily tasks, akin to a pianist practicing scales, the brain hones the specific neural circuits involved in those activities, making them stronger and more efficient.

- **Neurological Mechanisms of Recovery:**
  - **Synaptic Plasticity**:
    - Just like strengthening a muscle through weightlifting, synaptic plasticity involves reinforcing the connections between neurons, making the transmission of messages more efficient with every practice.

- **Cortical Reorganization**:
 - Picture a business reallocating its resources to different departments after a shock; the brain similarly reassigns functions from damaged to healthy areas, optimizing its resources for recovery.
- **Neurochemical Modulation**:
 - Parallel to a plant receiving nourishment, the brain adjusts neurotransmitter levels, including growth factors that foster neuron health, aiding recovery and growth.

Each of these therapies provides a scaffold for the brain's natural regenerative capabilities, prompting advancements in both motor and cognitive domains post-stroke. By targeting and stimulating specific neural pathways, these therapies leverage the brain's plastic nature, charting a course for far-reaching and sustained improvement in stroke aftermath. These insights not only advance our grasp of the brain's resilience but also highlight the potential for continuing recovery and adaptation in the face of adversity.

Grasping the principles of neuroplasticity opens the door to reimagining how we learn and teach. When educators understand the brain's ability to form and strengthen neural connections with the right stimulation, they can create learning experiences that are not only more engaging but also more effective. For instance, interactive and adaptive learning platforms, designed to evolve in response to a student's progress, mirror the way the brain strengthens pathways that are frequently traveled.

Advancements in technology, such as virtual reality and augmented reality, offer immersive experiences that could significantly enhance the learning process. Imagine history lessons where students can virtually walk through ancient cities or science classes where they can manipulate molecular structures in three dimensions—these are not just enthralling prospects, but they also capitalize on the brain's capacity for spatial and experiential learning.

Furthermore, neurofeedback, which allows individuals to see and modify their neural activity in real-time, is like giving learners a dashboard for their own brain. With this technology, they could learn to hone their focus and decrease stress, optimizing brain function for better learning outcomes.

All these approaches stand on the foundation of neuroplasticity, representing a shift from passive to active and personalized learning. They acknowledge that like a skilled athlete adjusts their training to optimize performance, students can tailor their learning strategies to strengthen their mental faculties, making the most of their brain's dynamic nature.

Let's take a closer look at how modern educational technologies finely weave the principles of neuroplasticity into the fabric of learning:

- **Interactive and Adaptive Learning Platforms:**
    - These platforms are powered by algorithms that adjust content in real-time, much like a skilled coach who changes the game plan based on an athlete's performance. By continuously assessing a student's responses, they tailor the difficulty and style of learning materials, ensuring that the brain is being challenged just enough to foster growth without causing frustration.
    - Neural engagement is front and center here; these platforms encourage active recall, critical thinking, and problem-solving, engaging a broad network of cognitive processes from memory to analytical skills, helping to solidify knowledge and build mental agility.

- **Virtual Reality (VR) and Augmented Reality (AR):**
    - VR and AR technologies immerse learners in a sensory-rich environment, not unlike an actor stepping into a convincing stage set. This multi-sensory engagement means that learners aren't just passively absorbing information but experiencing it, which can lead to stronger and more enduring neural connections.
    - Long-term retention and the practical application of knowledge are significantly impacted by these technologies. It's akin to a pilot using a flight simulator; by practicing in a realistic, controlled environment, the lessons learned are not only remembered more thoroughly but are also more easily translated into real-world skills.

- **Neurofeedback:**
    - Neurofeedback is like looking into a mirror that reflects your mental states. This technology provides real-time information about brainwave patterns, allowing individuals to learn how to modulate their focus, stress, and emotional responses. It trains the brain much in the way one hones the ability to meditate, refining attention and self-regulation.
    - Observing one's brain activity can heighten self-awareness and facilitate cognitive control, creating a feedback loop where the brain is learning about itself, encouraging a metacognitive approach to personal development.

In the broader landscape, empirical evidence supports the effectiveness of these technologies. Studies have shown enhanced engagement levels, improved academic performance, and greater retention of information among learners who use them. By integrating these applications into education systems, we are not only expanding the horizons of how knowledge is delivered but also tapping into the immense plasticity of the human brain, setting the stage for a future where learning is as dynamic and diverse as the brains we aim to educate.

In conclusion, our journey through the chapter has revealed the brain's extraordinary capacity for neuroplasticity. This feature of our neural architecture allows for continual growth and adaptation, akin to a software system that can update and refine its own code. It equips us with the power to overcome challenges, learn from a spectrum of experiences, and recover from injuries. Reflecting on this attribute of the brain should instill hope and a sense of empowerment in us all. We possess an in-built potential for transformation and resilience that can be harnessed at any age and stage of life, opening pathways to not only survive but thrive. This understanding should inspire us to engage with our brain's dynamic nature actively, embracing lifelong learning and adaptation.

STIMULATING THE PLASTIC BRAIN

Plasticity enables us to learn from the cradle to the grave, shaping our abilities, behaviors, and even our personalities. It underscores the brain's integral role in how we interact with the world, reinforcing the notion that our mental capacities are not fixed but are instead capable of extraordinary change. This transformative potential of our neural landscapes ensures that no matter the stage of life we are in, there is always room for growth, adaptation, and healing. Herein lies the foundation upon which we can build stronger, healthier, and more resilient minds.

Neuroplasticity rests on the interconnected workings of neurons, the brain's building blocks, and synapses, the junctions where neurons transmit signals to one another. Just as you might tighten the rigging in a ship to ensure the sails catch the wind more effectively, synaptic connections can be reinforced with repeated activity. This process is vital for learning and memory; each time you practice a skill or absorb new information, your brain reacts by strengthening the synaptic connections involved, making it easier to perform that action or recall that information in the future. It's a bit like creating a shortcut on your computer's desktop – the more you use it, the more efficient and accessible it becomes. This repetition is a fundamental principle of neuroplasticity, highlighting the importance of consistent practice and exposure when learning something new or trying to retain information.

Neurons, the cells that make up the brain, communicate with each other at junctions called synapses. When a neuron is active, it releases chemicals known as neurotransmitters into the synaptic space. These neurotransmitters cross the space and bind to receptors on the neighboring neuron, like a key fitting into a lock. This triggers a response in the receiving neuron, allowing the signal to continue its journey.

When this process repeats—whether through learning a new concept or practicing a skill—it leads to synaptic strengthening. It's similar to creating a well-worn path in a meadow by walking the same route repeatedly. The synapses become more efficient at transmitting signals, and the neuronal pathways involved in the task become more developed.

A significant player in this process is the protein Brain-Derived Neurotrophic Factor (BDNF). BDNF supports the survival of neurons and encourages the growth of new synapses, akin to a fertilizer that promotes the growth of plants. Learning stimulates the production of BDNF, enhancing the brain's ability to modify and strengthen synaptic connections.

Repeatedly practicing a task increases BDNF levels and activates these strengthened synaptic pathways, making the actions involved in that task become smoother and thought processes quicker. Over time, what may have once been a challenge becomes second nature, much like driving a familiar route without needing to consciously navigate each turn.

Through consistent repetition, neural pathways become more efficient, leading to mastery in a skill or the solidification of a memory. This is the fundamental mechanism underlying learning and long-term memory retention, a testament to the adaptive power of the brain and its ability to cultivate growth and change throughout life.

Think of the brain as the ultimate high-performance engine. It's the power behind your every thought, decision, and movement. But like any sophisticated engine, its performance heavily depends on the quality of its fuel and maintenance. Good nutrition fuels the brain with premium energy, much as high-octane fuel propels a race car around the track with efficiency and speed. Hydration acts as the cooling system, preventing overheating and keeping everything running smoothly, while a lack of water can cause the brain to sputter and stall.

Adequate sleep is the equivalent of routine maintenance; during sleep, the brain performs crucial repairs and clearing out waste, similar to how a car undergoes servicing to keep it in optimal condition. Without enough rest, the brain, like an overworked engine, can experience wear and tear that impairs its ability to function.

Even the "oil" of the brain — hormones and neurotransmitters — can affect its working. Stress, for instance, can introduce grit into the gears, wearing down the system, whereas relaxation and positive experiences keep the gears shifting smoothly.

In this way, lifestyle choices act as either performance enhancers or inhibitors to our brain's complex inner workings, directly influencing our cognitive horsepower and driving the quality of our mental acuity and agility.

Let's take a deeper look at the nourishment of the brain, likening it to premium fuel that enhances a car's performance. Omega-3 fatty acids act as a high-grade fuel, facilitating the building of cellular structures in the brain, including neurons and synapses. Just as clean fuel keeps a car's engine running without hiccups, omega-3s ensure the brain's messaging system is fluid and uninterrupted. Antioxidants, akin to an engine's air filter, protect the brain's delicate tissues by combating oxidative stress that can otherwise 'gunk up' the works. Amino acids serve as the specialized mechanics, repairing and maintaining neurotransmitters which dictate mood, energy, and focus.

Turning to sleep, think of non-REM and REM stages as a car's overnight servicing. Non-REM sleep lays down the groundwork for memory consolidation, similar to a mechanic arranging the tools and parts needed for the repair work. Then comes REM sleep, which is like the car's deep-cleaning process where waste products are removed and the system is fine-tuned. This ensures that what we've learned during the day is 'installed' properly, and our brain is refreshed for new information.

Stress hormones like cortisol can be compared to a car's alarm system. In moderate amounts, it's essential for alert responses, but when it's blaring incessantly, it can wear down the system, leading to cognitive 'engine' fatigue. On the flip side, neurotransmitters like serotonin and dopamine are the oil and lubricants, ensuring the gears of our thought processes shift smoothly and efficiently without overheating. Balancing these chemical elements is as crucial as maintaining the right mixture of oils in a car engine to prevent corrosion and ensure peak operation.

Through this analogy, we can see how integral it is to provide our brains with the right 'maintenance' and 'fuels' to facilitate peak cognitive performance and long-term health.

Regular physical activity is like a tune-up for your brain, ensuring it runs smoothly and efficiently. Exercise increases heart rate, which pumps more oxygen to the brain. It also aids the release of hormones that provide an excellent environment for the growth of brain cells.

Aerobic exercises like jogging, swimming, or cycling are particularly effective. They act as endurance training for the brain, improving both the structure and function of crucial regions linked to memory and learning. Strength training, though less studied, has also been shown to boost cognitive function, possibly by stimulating the release of growth factors that encourage neuronal health.

High-intensity interval training (HIIT) adds another layer, akin to performance boosting in cars, by providing short, sharp bursts of activity that challenge the brain and body in unique ways. Meanwhile, activities that require coordination, such as dance or team sports, not only work the body but also sharpen the mind by requiring complex motor skills and strategic thinking.

Flexibility exercises, such as yoga, emphasize steady breathing and require sustained attention, which can help improve the brain's connectivity and stress resilience. Together, these various forms of exercise compound their benefits, creating a well-rounded regimen for brain health that helps maintain cognitive function and emotional well-being. It's clear that staying physically active is integral to supporting a strong and capable brain throughout life.

Here is the breakdown on how different types of exercises bolster brain function, each serving as a specialized training program for your neural circuits:

- **Aerobic Exercises:**
  - **The release of neurotrophins and improved neurogenesis:**
    - Just like a car engine getting a burst of high-quality fuel, aerobic exercise floods the brain with substances that promote the birth of new neurons, especially in the hippocampus, an area critical for memory.
  - **Enhancement of synaptic plasticity and increased cerebral blood flow:**
    - Aerobic activities ramp up blood flow, akin to enhancing the oil flow in an engine for smoother operation, ensuring that the brain's connections are well-nourished and ready to rewire as needed.
  - **Specific effects on the hippocampus and prefrontal cortex:**
    - Imagine the hippocampus and prefrontal cortex as the brain's

command center; aerobic exercise strengthens this control hub, enhancing memory and decision-making.

- **Strength Training:**
  - **Release of growth factors like BDNF and IGF-1:**
    - Weightlifting leads to the release of BDNF and IGF-1, compounds that act as the brain's restorative agents, repairing and strengthening neural connections.
  - **Impact on brain structure, including white matter integrity:**
    - Much like reinforcing the framework of a building, strength training helps maintain and improve the brain's white matter, which is crucial for efficient communication between brain regions.
  - **Cognitive benefits observed in working memory and executive functions:**
    - Regular strength training can boost the brain's 'muscle memory' and sharpen our ability to plan and solve problems.

- **High-Intensity Interval Training (HIIT):**
  - **Acute effects on neurotransmitter release and neural excitability:**
    - HIIT sessions trigger a rapid release of neurotransmitters, akin to revving the engine, which can increase neural activity and readiness for learning.
  - **Chronic adaptations in cognitive function with regular HIIT:**
    - Over time, like tuning a car for optimal performance, HIIT can lead to improvements in attention span, processing speed, and even creativity.

- **Coordination Exercises (Dance, Team Sports):**
  - **Improvements in motor skills and spatial memory:**
    - Engaging in dance or sports is like running a complex software on a computer, enhancing the brain's ability to coordinate movement and spatial awareness.
  - **Neurological effects of complex movements and social interaction:**
    - These activities provide dual benefits: the physical demand of complex movement and the cognitive engagement from social interactions, both of which sharpen overall brain function.

- **Flexibility Exercises (Yoga):**
  - **The role of breathing and attention in modulating the autonomic

nervous system:
- Yoga requires focused breathing, which can calm the 'idle' of the brain, much like a smooth idling engine, leading to better stress management.
- **Stress reduction and its protective effects on the brain:**
- Committing to a routine of flexibility exercises reinforces the brain's resilience, much like a protective finish on a car, shielding against the wear and tear of daily stressors.

Understanding the connection between these physical activities and brain health enables us to see our workouts not just as a means to improve our physical stamina and strength, but also as vital maintenance for our cognitive functions, ensuring our minds remain as fit and agile as our bodies.

Tackling a jigsaw puzzle or diving into a new language is to your brain what lifting weights is to your muscles. Just as biceps become more defined with each curl, neural connections grow stronger and more efficient with each new word memorized or problem solved. These mental gymnastics induce a process called synaptic plasticity, which, in the gym analogy, is like increasing muscle fiber recruitment over time. Not only does this mental strength training enhance current cognitive capacity, but it also erects a robust scaffolding for future learning and brain health, much as consistent physical exercise fortifies the body against injury and decline. Engaging regularly in such brain-challenging activities ensures that the mind stays sharp, adaptable, and ready to tackle any complex task at hand, mirroring the satisfaction and benefits of a well-rounded, consistent gym routine.

Here is the breakdown on the cognitive strengthening that occurs when you engage in mental exercises like puzzles and learning new languages:

- <u>**Mental Exercises:**</u>
  - **Enhancement of neurogenesis:**
    - Think of each new cognitive challenge as a workout that not only flexes existing brain cells but also encourages the growth of new ones, expanding the brain's capacity.
  - **Synaptic Plasticity:**
    - **Long-term potentiation:**
      - Much like how using a muscle repeatedly makes it stronger, engaging in mental exercises regularly makes synapses more robust, facilitating quicker and stronger connections.
    - **Neural efficiency:**
      - Just like carving out a well-defined path through a dense forest,

mental exercises hone neural pathways, allowing for faster and more efficient information processing.

- **Cognitive Benefits:**
    - **Executive function:**
    - Working through challenges enhances the brain's command center, much like a director smoothly running a complex play, leading to sharper problem-solving and decision-making skills.
    - **Memory retention:**
    - Engaging with puzzles or new vocabulary stabilizes and consolidates memories, akin to repeatedly saving a file to ensure it's not lost or corrupted.
    - **Language acquisition:**
    - Learning a new language engages multiple brain regions, fostering new connections in the brain's network – it's like setting up a sophisticated communication system that boosts all aspects of cognitive function.

Just as resistance training promotes muscle growth and endurance, mental exercises build up the brain's strength and resilience. By regularly challenging the brain with new and complex tasks, you are, in essence, equipping it with the agility to navigate an ever-changing environment, underscoring the vital role of cognitive exercises in the development of a strong and adaptable mind.

Stress, a familiar visitor to most, can play a dual role in the brain's plasticity, acting as both a hindrance and a catalyst. In the face of immediate, short-lived stress, the brain's plasticity is enhanced, allowing for a quick response to challenges—much like a sprinter's muscles springing into action. However, chronic stress is another story. It can flood the brain with stress hormones like cortisol, which, over time, can wear down the brain's ability to form new connections, akin to a machine grinding to a halt from overuse.

To mitigate these effects, various stress reduction techniques can be employed. Mindfulness meditation, for instance, acts as a pressure valve, releasing the build-up of stress and restoring the brain's plasticity. Regular physical exercise is another effective technique, clearing the mental cobwebs and rejuvenating the mind's capacity for change and adaptation. Adequate sleep, social interaction, and hobbies can also play significant roles in buffering the brain against the erosive effects of long-term stress.

By understanding and implementing these strategies, we can protect and enhance our brain's malleability. Addressing stress is not just about feeling better in the moment; it's about protecting our brain's long-term health and functionality, ultimately shaping our ability to learn, adapt, and thrive in an ever-changing environment.

Let's take a closer look at the intricate dance between stress and the brain, and how various techniques can tip the scales towards a healthier, more plastic mind:

- **Physiological Impacts of Stress:**
  - **Cortisol release and its effect on synaptic plasticity:**
    - Picture cortisol as a floodgate. When stress hits, the gates open and cortisol flows through the brain, initially sharpening our senses and memory. However, prolonged exposure can oversaturate the brain, dampening the formation of new connections and the brain's ability to reorganize itself – much like a flooded engine struggling to run.
  - **Inflammatory pathways activated by chronic stress:**
    - Chronic stress can light a slow-burning fire within the brain's immune system, leading to inflammation that can slowly erode the brain's structure, akin to rust on a car's undercarriage.
  - **Impacts on the hippocampus and memory under stress:**
    - The hippocampus, the brain's memory center, can shrink under constant stress, akin to a database losing storage space, making it harder to save and retrieve memories.

- **Stress Reduction Techniques:**
  - **Mindfulness Meditation:**
    - Engaging in mindfulness is like bringing in a skilled technician to recalibrate the brain's stress response. It coaxes brain regions involved in focus and emotions to settle into a more harmonious rhythm, while the amygdala – the brain's alarm system – quietens, reducing its knee-jerk reactions to stress.
  - **Physical Exercise:**
    - Exercise boosts the production of BDNF, a substance that repairs and protects brain cells, much like a restorative oil treatment for an engine. It also acts like a thermostat, regulating the stress response so the brain doesn't overheat from excessive cortisol.
  - **Adequate Sleep:**
    - Quality sleep acts as an overnight cleanup crew for the brain. It prunes unnecessary connections, much like trimming away dead branches to allow a

tree to flourish, and fortifies the pathways we rely on, keeping our memory recall sharp and efficient.
- **Social Interaction and Hobbies:**
- Socializing and pursuing hobbies inject the brain with a sense of purpose and joy, much like customizing a car can enhance its performance and the driver's connection to it. These activities ward off perceived stress and promote a nimble, resilient mind.

Through these analogies, we see how counteracting stress with targeted strategies not only helps us feel more at ease but also catalyzes the brain's adaptive abilities – ensuring it remains a high-performance machine capable of learning, growing, and navigating the twists and turns of life.

Neuroplasticity, the brain's ability to rewire itself, is not just a theoretical concept but a real phenomenon that can lead to remarkable cognitive transformations. Barbara Arrowsmith-Young, for instance, reshaped her own learning disabilities into unique strengths by developing brain exercises that leveraged neuroplasticity. Similarly, individuals who have suffered strokes have managed to recover abilities that were once thought permanently lost. By employing tailored rehabilitation programs focused on repetitive and targeted exercises, these individuals retrained different brain areas to take over lost functions, showcasing the brain's incredible capacity to adapt and heal. These stories of personal cognitive triumphs are the ultimate testament to the brain's malleability and the potential for positive change, regardless of age or condition. They remind us that with dedication and the right strategies, overcoming neurological challenges is within reach.

Mindfulness is a straightforward yet potent practice with roots in ancient meditation traditions, now backed by modern science as a technique that reinforces neuroplasticity. In essence, mindfulness involves paying focused attention to the present moment, often starting with the breath. It's like training a microscope on your own mind, observing without judgment. This practice is thought to strengthen the brain's ability to concentrate and can lead to structural changes in regions associated with attention, emotion regulation, and self-awareness.

Engaging in regular mindfulness exercises, such as guided or silent meditation, can be comparable to a workout regimen for the brain. It doesn't require equipment or significant time investment but rather a consistent, dedicated approach. By setting aside a few minutes daily, individuals can potentially enhance their cognitive flexibility, reduce stress responses, and improve their overall mental well-being.

The sequential steps of mindfulness—such as focusing on the breath, noticing when the mind wanders, and gently returning to the breath—train the brain's 'muscles' for focus and calm. Over time, just like muscles become stronger and more defined with regular exercise, so too does the brain develop a heightened capacity for mindful awareness, which can spill over positively into all aspects of life.

Here is the breakdown of how mindfulness practice promotes neurological and cognitive enhancements, much like cultivating a flourishing garden improves its biodiversity and resilience:

- **Neurological Changes:**
  - **Structural alterations in the prefrontal cortex:**
    - Similar to bolstering the foundation of a house, mindfulness can increase the gray matter density in the prefrontal cortex, the brain's decision-making and personality hub.
    - This results in enhanced connections between brain regions, akin to upgrading the wiring in a home to improve electricity flow and appliance function.
  - **Impact on the amygdala:**
    - Mindfulness can effectively shrink the amygdala, our built-in security system, leading to improved stress regulation like installing a more sophisticated alarm system that discriminates real threats from false alarms.
    - It modulates the fight or flight response, making it less likely to hit the panic button during minor stress, similar to how a well-trained guard assesses situations more calmly.
  - **Changes in the anterior cingulate cortex (ACC):**
    - Strengthening the ACC through mindfulness is like fine-tuning a car's steering for better control and navigation, leading to improved self-regulation and error detection.
    - The heightened cognitive flexibility is akin to an athlete developing a broader range of motion, allowing for superior adaptation and skill execution.

- **Cognitive Improvements:**
  - **Attention and Concentration:**
    - Mindfulness stabilizes attention, much like a tripod steadies a camera for a clear shot. It helps maintain focus and clarity, even amidst distractions.
    - It plays a vital role in preventing attentional lapses, similar to a vigilant

lifeguard who keeps watch over swimmers, ensuring that one's mental resources are attentively guarding against mind-wandering.
- **Emotion Regulation:**
- Mindfulness is akin to a skilled negotiator, helping to manage emotions more effectively and reducing the intensity and duration of negative emotional episodes.
- The practice improves emotional reactivity and recovery, equipping individuals with rapid cooldown mechanisms like those in an advanced computer system.
- **Self-Awareness:**
- Enhancing introspection and self-knowledge with mindfulness is like upgrading a car's GPS for better navigation through one's mental landscape.
- The benefits of increased self-awareness span across daily life, improving interpersonal skills and decision-making, much like improved visibility aids in safer driving.

By regularly engaging in mindfulness practices and reaping these benefits, individuals can fortify their mental terrain, ensuring that their cognitive capabilities remain robust, adaptable, and prepared for life's challenges and opportunities.

Neuroplasticity endows us with the potential for lifelong learning and mental growth. This innate capability of our brains to form and reorganize synaptic connections in response to experiences lays the groundwork for us to improve our cognitive abilities, recover from brain injuries, and adapt to new challenges. Embracing a proactive stance towards brain health can significantly influence our quality of life, as it empowers us to continually develop and refine our skills and behaviors. By engaging in activities that stimulate neuroplasticity, such as learning new skills, practicing mindfulness, and maintaining a healthy lifestyle, we can harness this remarkable adaptability for personal development and well-being. The implications for education, rehabilitation, and overall human potential are vast, positioning neuroplasticity not just as a scientific fact, but as a beacon of hope for anyone looking to enhance their cognitive capabilities and lead a fulfilling life.

NEUROPLASTICITYS DARK SIDE

Neuroplasticity, while fundamentally the brain's impressive capability to adapt and evolve, can have a downside. The same processes that allow us to acquire skills and recover from injuries can also lead to persistent, undesirable behaviors. Think of the brain as having a system of roads: when you learn something new or change your behavior, you build new roads, and the more you travel on them, the wider and more permanent they become. Similarly, in the realm of neuroplasticity, repeated thoughts or actions reinforce certain neural pathways, strengthening their influence on behavior.

This becomes problematic when the reinforced pathways are maladaptive, such as those developed through drug use or other harmful habits. Every time a person indulges in these behaviors, their brain further paves and broadens these neural "roads," making it increasingly challenging to travel any differently. It's like a city where the main roads lead to an unsafe district, and despite the dangers, it's where all the traffic flows because the roads are so well-developed.

This concept can be tough to navigate for the amateur mind. But by breaking down the brain's complex network into understandable roadmaps, we can see how negative patterns are formed and maintained. It also reveals potential strategies to build new, healthier pathways — akin to constructing new roads that lead to better destinations. In this chapter, we'll guide you through the intricate web of neuroplasticity's less favorable roles and how they affect us, pondering both the causes of these detrimental patterns and applicable ways to overcome them.

When we repeat certain behaviors, our brain begins to solidify these actions into habits through a process called synaptic strengthening. Here's a step-by-step guide to how this works and how to form more positive habits:

1. **Reinforcement of Neural Pathways**: Each time you perform an action, your neurons communicate by sending signals across synapses. Neurotransmitters like dopamine are released, which can lead to a feeling of

reward. If the action is repeated, this synaptic transmission becomes more efficient, forging a stronger neural pathway. It's like carving a deeper groove on a dirt road every time a vehicle passes.

2. **Role of Neurotransmitters in Addiction**: Addictive substances or behaviors lead to an exaggerated release of neurotransmitters, creating a powerful sense of reward. With addiction, this reward system becomes hijacked, and the synaptic connections related to the substance or behavior become stronger, making it more difficult to resist. Essentially, the brain begins to prioritize these harmful activities over healthier choices.

3. **Cognitive-Behavioral Therapy (CBT)**: To combat addiction or maladaptive behaviors, CBT can be employed as mental 'cognitive roadwork.' This therapy works by helping individuals recognize harmful thought patterns and actively change their behaviors. It's like replacing old, damaged roads with new ones that lead to better destinations.

4. **Creating New Neural Pathways**: To establish a new, healthy habit, it involves repeated practice of the desired behavior. It's similar to paving a new road through consistent effort. Over time, this road becomes more prominent and easier to travel.

5. **Consistent Practice and Environmental Changes**: Just as city planners would create environments to promote smoother traffic flow, developing an environment that supports your new habits is crucial. This could be by avoiding triggers for harmful behaviors or adding reminders for positive ones. Consistency is key, much like keeping up with road maintenance to avoid potholes.

6. **Maintenance of New Habits**: Maintain these new behaviors by continually reinforcing these pathways, akin to frequent travel on a new road to keep it well-trodden and accessible, ensuring that the alternative, less healthy paths, become overgrown and less traveled.

By understanding these steps and persistently applying cognitive strategies, we can begin to steer our neuroplasticity towards a realm of improvement and sustained health. It's a testament to our ability to change and adapt, even in the face of challenging, deep-rooted behaviors.

Just like a well-trodden path through a forest becomes easier to navigate over time, our brain solidifies behaviors through repetition, creating easy-to-follow neural tracks. When we practice playing the piano daily or jog every morning, our brain lays down pathways that make it easier to repeat these actions. It's like using a machete to clear a path in a dense jungle; the more you travel it, the clearer and more defined it becomes.

Conversely, if we fall into a daily routine of less constructive behaviors, such as smoking or procrastinating, our brain also reinforces these paths, making them hard to break away from. Imagine every time you take a shortcut through a grassy field, the grass gets trampled down more and more until a visible path forms, beckoning you to use it again and again.

As simple as it is to form a habit, the type of habit—beneficial or harmful—depends on the actions we choose to repeat. Recognizing this, we can take deliberate strides in laying down pathways that lead to better health, relationships, and overall well-being, just as a city planner carefully designs roads to improve the flow of traffic and ease of travel for its inhabitants.

Let's take a deeper look at how habits carve their signature into the brain's landscape. Imagine your neural pathways as streets in a bustling city. Each time you engage in a behavior, it's like sending a car down a particular street. The more cars you send, the more the road is used, and the more likely you are to keep using it. That's your brain, building a superhighway for this repeated action through a process called synaptic strengthening.

Now, let's talk about the neurotransmitter dopamine, which plays a role similar to a city's traffic lights. It signals when it's time to 'go'—in the brain's case, providing a feel-good reward that encourages you to repeat the behavior. Dopamine reinforces the pathway, making the 'street' more prominent with each pass, leading to a stronger synaptic connection.

When the behavior is something positive, like regular exercise, these reinforced pathways enhance well-being—equivalent to bustling trade routes that bring prosperity to city areas. But when the behavior is negative, such as smoking, these neural pathways can lead to areas of ill health—like roads that lead to a polluted, rundown district.

If you want to change a habit, you need to build a new road and redirect the traffic. This is where cognitive strategies come in. Techniques such as CBT are like urban development initiatives for the brain. They help construct new routes by practicing alternative behaviors, and, with consistent effort, these can become the preferred pathways, much like a new highway eases congestion by offering a better path.

To maintain these new routes, changes in the environment—like removing ashtrays or unhealthy snacks from your home—can help divert traffic from the old path to the new. It's comparable to adding amenities that attract more people to a revitalized urban area, solidifying its popularity.

Understanding this dynamic process, we gain the tools not just to comprehend but to direct the constant construction of our brain's pathways. Every choice we make is a brushstroke on the vast canvas of our minds, and with care, we can ensure the picture that emerges is one of health and happiness. Let these insights into the brain's workings empower you to lay down neural paths that lead to the very best versions of yourself.

In real-life scenarios, the principle of neuroplasticity can unwittingly foster detrimental behaviors, such as in the case of addiction. For instance, someone who begins using drugs or alcohol as a coping mechanism can find over time that their brain's circuitry has adapted to this behavior. The neurotransmitter dopamine plays a crucial role here; it's released in large quantities during drug use, reinforcing the desire to continue using due to the intense sense of reward it triggers.

This neurochemical process creates a loop. The brain, now accustomed to the dopamine surge, strengthens the neural pathways associated with substance use, effectively 'learning' this behavior. It's similar to someone learning to drive the same route every day until it becomes automatic, except in this case, the destination is harmful.

Persistent activities like prolonged stress, negative thinking, or unhealthy eating patterns can similarly sculpt neural pathways that lead to anxiety, depression, or obesity. These patterns become the brain's default, making it increasingly challenging to adopt healthier strategies or thought processes without intentional intervention.

Connecting these real-life cases back to neuroplasticity's impacts, it's clear that while the brain's adaptability is extraordinary, it does not distinguish between beneficial and harmful behaviors in its tendency to solidify repeated actions into habits. Recognizing this allows us to identify harmful patterns and work towards redirecting our brain's plasticity into more positive tracks, akin to rerouting a river's flow to foster a more fertile landscape.

Here is the breakdown of how persistent negative behaviors solidify in the brain and the actionable strategies to undo these patterns:

- **Neural Pathway Entrenchment:**
  - **Chronology of habit formation:**
    - Just as footprints form a path in soft soil, repeated actions leave neural imprints in the brain, which over time create well-defined paths or habits.
  - **The role of dopamine in reinforcing the habit loop:**
    - Imagine dopamine like a signpost that rewards the brain each time it travels down a particular path, encouraging it to take that route again.
  - **Neurochemical changes resulting from repeated behaviors:**
    - As actions are repeated, the neurotransmitter activity strengthens the associations, much like rain hardens the soil on a frequently used path, making it more permanent.

- **Negative Habit Formation:**
  - **Step-by-step process from initiation to routine:**
    - Negative behaviors start as shortcuts to reward or relief, becoming ingrained routes in the brain's landscape through continued use.
  - **Cognitive and emotional repercussions:**
    - These negative patterns can cloud judgment and fuel a cycle of negative emotions, resembling a smog that affects the entire city's atmosphere.
  - **Physiological changes in the brain:**
    - The brain physically adapts to support these destructive behaviors, akin to a city developing infrastructure that unfortunately promotes unhealthy living.

- **Reversal Strategies:**
  - **Identification and interruption of negative habits:**
    - Pinpoint these habits like identifying faulty wiring in a complex circuit and then cutting it off to prevent further damage.

- **Replacement with positive behaviors:**
  - Introduce new behaviors, like building new roads in a city, which provide alternate, healthier routes for traffic flow.
- **Long-term reinforcement of new habits:**
  - Consistent practice strengthens these pathways, similar to how a newly constructed road becomes more widely used as people become aware of it.

By approaching this transformation step by step, you can gradually reshape your brain's pathways. It's like renovating a city, making it cleaner, more efficient, and healthier for all its inhabitants. Cognitive-behavioral techniques serve as the tools for this renovation, helping to methodically dismantle the old and build up the new, facilitating a fresh pattern of thought and behavior that fosters a better quality of life.

Rewiring the brain to break free from negative patterns is akin to reprogramming a misfiring circuit. Imagine an electrician who locates a faulty wire that's causing a short circuit. They don't just remove the wire; they replace it with one that's properly insulated and reroute it to ensure the electricity flows safely and efficiently. Similarly, when we want to change a bad habit, we need to identify the 'faulty' neural pathways our brains have been using. We then intentionally create new pathways through repeated, positive behavior—like laying down new wiring that reroutes our thoughts and actions.

Think also of a ship's captain steering their vessel away from perilous waters. If the ship has been sailing on a risky path, the captain doesn't just jerk the wheel; they chart a new, safer course and follow it consistently until it becomes familiar. In the same way, adopting new behaviors and thought patterns requires us to set a fresh course and stick to it until our brain automatically follows this better path.

By consistently practicing alternative behaviors and reinforcing them, we can rewire our brains, laying down new pathways that become our new 'default' settings. It's not an overnight fix; it's a journey that takes patience, persistence, and a steady hand on the wheel, but with time, we can navigate our brains towards healthier behaviors and thought processes, reshaping our lives along the way.

To reshape our brain's circuitry for more positive habits, we follow a methodical guide that mirrors the work an electrician might perform on a misfiring electrical circuit, or the careful planning of a ship's journey to avoid treacherous waters.

1. **Identify the Negative Pattern:** Begin by recognizing the habits that are akin to faulty wires in our brain's circuitry. These are the behaviors or thoughts that short-circuit our success or well-being.

2. **Disconnect the Old Pathway:** Like an electrician who turns off the power to repair wiring, take deliberate steps to interrupt the negative habits. This could mean altering routines, avoiding triggers, or consciously implementing counter-actions.

3. **Lay Down New Wiring:** Just as an electrician lays down new, safe wiring, start forming new neural pathways with positive, constructive behaviors. This might mean practicing mindfulness instead of reaching for a cigarette, or going for a walk when feeling the urge to procrastinate.

4. **Reinforce the New Pathway:** To ensure that the new behaviors stick, they must be practiced consistently. Like reinforcing the foundations of a well-built road or repeatedly following a successful sea route, this repetition strengthens the new neural connections.

5. **Navigate Challenges:** Anticipate the challenges that will inevitably arise, much like a ship captain who plans for storms. Arm yourself with strategies to overcome these challenges, such as having a support system or reminding yourself of the long-term benefits of your new habits.

6. **Persistence and Adaptation:** Maintaining the new pathway requires perseverance. Just as an electrician must test and retest their work, or a ship must adapt its route based on the weather conditions, you will need to refine your strategies and keep at them, even when it's tough.

7. **Monitor Progress and Adjust:** Finally, similar to how an electrician would monitor a newly repaired circuit over time or a navigator would revise their charts, keep track of your progress and be ready to adjust your approach

to continue avoiding the 'faults' and sailing smoothly.

With patience and persistence, these steps can lead to a rewiring of sorts - moving from the 'short circuits' of negative habits to the creation of a robust network of positive, healthy connections in the brain. This transformation is not immediate, but with careful and consistent effort, just like the work of a skilled electrician or a masterful captain, you can navigate your thought patterns towards safer, more fruitful shores.

Personal stories of recovery and transformation bear witness to the incredible adaptability of the human brain. Through neuroplasticity, individuals have managed to redirect their lives after suffering from debilitating habits or traumatic experiences. For example, stroke survivors have relearned to walk and speak, effectively rewriting their brain's damaged pathways through intensive therapy and practice. People with addictions have broken free from the chains of their dependencies by reinforcing healthier habits, reshaping their brain's reward system one day at a time. These accounts are not just anecdotes; they are evidence of neuroplasticity's central role in personal growth and recovery, demonstrating that with effort, support, and time, change is more than just a possibility—it's a reality grounded in the malleability of our brains.

Understanding neuroplasticity unlocks a powerful truth about our brains: they are designed to change and adapt. This knowledge is not simply academic; it carries the potential for profound personal transformation. By consciously engaging in activities that stimulate our minds, such as learning new skills, practicing mindfulness, or fostering positive relationships, we can deliberately influence our brain's plastic nature. It is a call to action to embrace a proactive stance in life, using the principles of neuroplasticity to craft a more fulfilling, healthier, and adaptable existence. It serves as an invitation to take control of our neurological destinies, harnessing the dynamic potential of our brains for the betterment of our lives and the communities we inhabit.

TECHNOLOGICAL ADVANCES AND NEUROPLASTICITY

Brain-computer interface (BCI) technology acts as a groundbreaking bridge linking the human mind's complex neural network with the vast digital realm. Picture a bridge spanning a river, connecting two bustling cities that, until now, had no direct way to communicate. On one side, we have the rich, organic world of human thoughts and emotions; on the other, the binary, calculated landscape of computers and the internet. BCI serves as the infrastructure that facilitates a two-way exchange of information, allowing thoughts to direct digital actions and digital feedback to influence neural activity.

Just as a physical bridge allows for the exchange of goods and ideas, enhancing the growth and interaction of societies on either side, BCI enables a direct dialogue between our brain and external devices. Imagine controlling a computer cursor with your thoughts or a prosthetic limb responding to neural commands—the potential and implications are profound. This technology not only expands the limits of human-machine interaction but also provides a powerful tool for learning and rehabilitation, fundamentally altering our brain's potential to adapt, recover, and evolve. It's a testament to human innovation, presenting new horizons for enhancing life and understanding the mysteries of the mind.

Here is the detailed breakdown of the core components of brain-computer interface technology, which bridges our cognitive processes with the capabilities of modern machines:

- **Signal Detection:**
  - **Types of brain signals targeted by BCI:**
    - Electrocorticographic (ECoG) signals, akin to the deep rumblings of an earthquake, conveying complex brain activity.
    - Electroencephalographic (EEG) signals, similar to the buzzing of a beehive, representing the collective output of millions of neurons.
  - **Methods used for signal detection and acquisition:**

- Non-invasive sensors placed on the scalp, like detectives listening for clues on the surface.
- Invasive electrodes implanted directly in the brain, capturing the whispers of individual neurons.

- **Signal Interpretation:**
  - **Algorithms for deciphering neural patterns:**
    - Complex software algorithms that act as translators, turning the Morse code of brain signals into a language that computers can understand.
  - **Translation of brain activity into commands:**
    - The interpreted signals are then turned into commands, much like a conductor turning sheet music into a symphony, orchestrating the actions of digital devices.

- **Command Execution:**
  - **Synchronization with external devices:**
    - A carefully timed dance between the brain's output and the device's response, ensuring they move together in harmony.
  - **Output mechanisms (e.g., movement in a prosthetic, cursor control):**
    - Resulting in actions as varied as a robotic arm painting a canvas or a digital cursor flying across a screen, all directed by the power of thought.

- **Feedback Loop:**
  - **How the brain receives and processes feedback from the BCI:**
    - Feedback is the brain's way of learning from the environment, like an echo returning to its source, allowing the individual to adjust and refine their control.
  - **The role of feedback in learning and neuroplastic adaptation:**
    - This continual feedback loop encourages the brain to adapt, similar to a musician tuning an instrument, refining the connection between neural intentions and digital outcomes.

By grasping each facet of BCI technology through these familiar comparisons, you can appreciate the sophistication behind a system that empowers the mind to extend its influence far beyond the physical limits of the body. This understanding is not merely technical but invites contemplation on the vast potential that such a union of brain and machine holds for the future of human capability.

In the evolving landscape of neuroscience, brain-computer interfaces (BCIs) stand out as a pivotal innovation. These systems enable a direct communication pipeline between the brain's electrical activity and computing devices. BCIs work by detecting signals from the brain, whether they are picked up non-invasively from the scalp or captured more directly via implanted electrodes. Algorithms then interpret these signals, translating neurological patterns into commands that machines can execute. This allows a person to control a computer cursor, for instance, using only their thoughts.

Feedback from the machine to the user is also critical. Just as you might adjust your movements based on what you see, BCIs provide visual, haptic, or auditory feedback, helping the brain fine-tune its outputs. This capability is not a one-way street; it's a dynamic loop where both entities—the biological and the technological—learn and adapt to each other.

This interactive loop has profound implications for fields like rehabilitation, where stroke survivors might retrain brain areas to compensate for lost functions, or in accessibility, offering individuals with mobility impairments new avenues to interact with the world. Here, BCI isn't just technology; it's a tool that reflects our ingenuity and adaptability, presenting new horizons in our ongoing dialogue with the digital world.

Let's take a closer look at the world of algorithms that underpins brain-computer interface (BCI) technology. Think of these algorithms as the skilled linguists of the computing world, translating the brain's complex neural language into clear, actionable instructions a machine can understand.

The first step in this intricate process is pattern recognition. Like identifying a bird from its song, the algorithm sifts through the brain's electrical symphony and pinpoints specific patterns that correspond to intended commands. These recognizable patterns are often amid a cacophony of neural noise, yet advanced signal processing techniques, akin to noise-cancelling headphones, allow the relevant information to be isolated and understood.

Error correction comes next, much like an editor polishes a draft, ensuring that the intended message is clear. The algorithm achieves this by comparing the brain's outputs against previously learned patterns, correcting deviations that might be mistakes. This ongoing refinement is critical; it ensures that the dialogue between the brain and the machine becomes increasingly fluent over time.

Moreover, the adaptability of these algorithms is akin to a conversation that becomes richer as both participants learn more about each other. Through machine learning techniques, BCIs evolve, improving their accuracy and responsiveness with each interaction. They make use of feedback, provided visually or through other senses, to let the brain know the outcome of its commands. This feedback is the equivalent of seeing a ball hit a target—informing the thrower of their accuracy and allowing them to adjust their aim on the next attempt.

The algorithms must also tackle the brain's variability—a feature as unique and changing as one's handwriting. Advanced neural decoding techniques enable the BCI to maintain consistency in interpretation, adjusting to the person's neural patterns as they shift through fatigue, focus, or even learning.

Altogether, these components work in harmony to grant users control over external devices, turning thoughts into action with precision and care. This is the prowess of BCI technology: a testament to human ingenuity and a beacon for future possibilities, where the boundaries between thought and action are seamlessly blurred.

Imagine neurofeedback as a personal brain coach, one that gives you real-time commentary on your mental performance. Just like a coach observing an athlete's form and providing instant feedback, neurofeedback mechanisms monitor your brain's electrical activity and present it in a way that you can understand. Using sensors, typically fitted to your head like a swim cap, the coach — or neurofeedback software — watches as your brain goes through its exercises, be it focusing or relaxing.

As you progress, the coach points out when you hit the bulls-eye, like when your focus sharpens and you feel that 'in the zone' sensation. It then guides you by showing you how often you're hitting the mark, and how you can adjust to improve, much like a batting coach that helps you fine-tune your swing based on where the ball lands. Over time, you learn to recognize the feeling of getting it right and can recreate it, even when the coach isn't watching — that's essentially your brain learning to regulate its own activity.

This continuous loop of action, observation, and adjustment trains your cognitive functions, ironing out the kinks in your mental processes. In the broader scheme of things, it means not just honing mental skills but also developing the capacity to manage emotions and reactions better, using nothing but your brain's own ability to adapt and optimize itself. Neurofeedback allows us to become the architects of our cognitive landscape, guiding us in a journey of personal mastery and mindfulness.

Here's the breakdown of the technologies and processes that make neurofeedback work, much like a complex dashboard brings a car's performance data to a driver's fingertips:

- **Types of Brain Waves Monitored:**
    - **Alpha waves for relaxation:** Picture these as the gentle rhythm of a calm sea, indicating a relaxed state of mind.
    - **Beta waves for alertness:** These are the choppy waves during a windy day, showing when we are alert and focused.
    - **Delta waves for deep sleep:** Imagine the deep ocean stillness, representing the restorative phase of deep sleep.

- **Neurofeedback Process:**
    - **Detection of brain wave patterns via sensors:** Like a weather station picking up signals from the atmosphere, these sensors detect the brain's electrical patterns.
    - **Analysis of wave patterns using specialized software:** This is the meteorologist interpreting the data, turning raw numbers into meaningful forecasts.
    - **Real-time visualization of brain activity for the user:** Think of this as a weather app on your phone, giving you an instant readout of your brain's conditions.

- **Feedback Types:**
    - **Visual:** Similar to watching the speedometer to maintain the right speed, visual feedback shows you how close your brain activity is to the desired state.
    - **Auditory:** Just as a musician tunes an instrument by ear, varying tones guide you toward the target brain wave state.
    - **Tactile:** This is like the vibration from a phone, a physical nudge indicating that your brain waves have hit the right note.

- **User Interaction:**
    - **How users learn to alter their brain waves through feedback:** It's akin to learning to ride a bike with balance feedback; you adjust your control based on the information received.
    - **Techniques for training attention, relaxation, or other cognitive states:** Consider this like practicing a golf swing, where subtle shifts and consistent practice lead to a perfect shot.

This process transforms the esoteric landscape of our brain's electrical activity into a user-friendly interface, empowering us to tune our mental state like a radio dial, finding the right station for our current needs. It's a confluence of precision technology and human experience that exemplifies how far we've come in understanding and harnessing the power of our own biology.

Neurofeedback has become a practical tool in various scenarios, offering a way for people to enhance cognitive function and control. In the case of individuals with ADHD, neurofeedback has been used as a training method to improve concentration and reduce impulsivity. By visualizing their brain activity in real-time, typically through computer games or displays that respond to their level of focus, these individuals can practice maintaining a state that resembles the calm and alertness needed for tasks requiring attention.

For athletes, neurofeedback serves a different purpose. It's used to fine-tune reactions and sharpen focus under pressure, much like a sprinter perfecting their start off the blocks. Athletes engage in exercises that train their brains to enter 'the zone,' a state of peak performance. By learning to regulate brainwaves associated with optimal focus and calm, they can perform better during competitions.

The clear, quantifiable feedback from neurofeedback sessions allows both individuals with ADHD and athletes to measure their progress. They can see when their brain is in the desired state, identify when it's not, and adjust accordingly. Over time, the goal is for these improved patterns of brain activity to become second nature, enhancing everyday life as well as specific tasks that require intense concentration and mental stability.

Neurofeedback training programs are designed to harness the brain's plasticity and improve cognitive function through tailored exercises. Here's a step-by-step guide on how these programs typically operate for ADHD patients and athletes, illustrating the meticulous process that underpins this cutting-edge therapy.

Step 1: **Assessment and Calibration**
Before starting, an initial assessment is conducted to understand the individual's brainwave patterns. This might involve recording the brain's electrical activity with an EEG during various tasks or while at rest. For ADHD patients, the focus is often on identifying signatures of inattention or impulsivity, whereas for athletes, it might be about pinpointing the brain waves associated with optimal focus and performance.

Step 2: **Selecting Neurofeedback Protocols**
Depending on the assessment, different neurofeedback protocols are chosen:
- For individuals with ADHD, protocols might aim to decrease theta waves (associated with drowsiness) and increase beta waves (associated with alertness).
- Athletes might use protocols to enhance alpha wave production for a calm focus or sensorimotor rhythm (SMR) training to improve motor control.

Step 3: **Targeting Specific Brain Regions**
Neurofeedback training is localized:
- ADHD protocols might target the prefrontal cortex, crucial for attention control.
- Athletes' training could be focused on the motor cortex or areas responsible for visual processing depending on their sport.

Step 4: **Undergoing Training Sessions**
During sessions, individuals interact with software that provides feedback based on their brain activity:
- ADHD patients may play a game that only progresses when they're in the correct brainwave state.
- Athletes might use a simulation that requires them to maintain focus to achieve higher scores.

Step 5: **Receiving Real-Time Feedback**
Feedback is given instantly during these activities, allowing participants to understand when they're successfully engaging the targeted brain waves:
- This feedback can be auditory, like a change in volume, or visual, like an on-screen meter.

Step 6: **Adapting the Training**
The neurofeedback equipment often includes adaptive algorithms that adjust the difficulty of the task in real-time based on performance.

Step 7: **Consolidating Neuroplastic Changes**
Repeated sessions facilitate neuroplastic changes over time, essentially rewiring the brain:
- ADHD patients might experience improved attention and reduced impulsivity as the brain learns to sustain an attentive state.
- Athletes may notice enhanced performance during high-pressure situations as their brains become adept at entering a state of flow more reliably.

Step 8: **Tracking and Analysis of Outcomes**
Progress is typically monitored throughout the training program, with ongoing assessments to evaluate improvements in cognitive and behavioral metrics relative to the goals set at the beginning.

Neurofeedback programs are carefully crafted to meet the needs of the individual, responding intelligently to the brain's unique patterns. By steadily guiding the brain towards optimal functioning, neurofeedback training lays the groundwork for lasting cognitive and performance enhancements, tailored to the demands of daily life and specific activities.

Virtual reality can be likened to a mental gymnasium. It's a place where, instead of lifting weights or running on treadmills, the brain is the one performing the workouts. With a VR headset, much like a pair of athletic shoes, you step into a digital space designed to strengthen mental muscles. Through immersive and interactive scenarios, the brain practices and hones skills such as memory, attention, and problem-solving.

Just as a gym is equipped with various stations for different exercises, virtual reality presents an array of environments and tasks—each crafted to target specific cognitive faculties. A memory challenge in VR might involve navigating a labyrinth, with each turn sharpening the brain's ability to recall and sequence information. An attention task might require tracking moving objects, training focus and concentration amidst digital distractions.

This form of mental training does more than just engage the brain; it immerses it in highly stimulative experiences that can reshape and enhance cognitive processes. And just like a personal trainer who assesses your physical performance and customizes your workout, VR programs can adapt to the level of challenge that you need, ensuring that the brain's training regimen is not only rigorous but also tailored to your personal growth trajectory.

Here is the breakdown of how virtual reality (VR) serves as a digital incubator for cognitive skills, akin to how a versatile playground stimulates a child's physical and mental growth:

- **Sensory Inputs in VR:**
  - **Visual:** VR immerses you in three-dimensional spaces as varied as the ecosystems on Earth. Puzzles may imitate intricate mazes found in nature, while games emulate the need to identify patterns and details, like distinguishing camouflaged animals in the wild.
  - **Auditory:** Sounds in VR direct attention or set a scene, much like how the rustle of leaves can signal an animal's approach or the change of a bird's song speaks to the time of day.
  - **Haptic:** Simulating touch, VR can mimic textures and resistance, offering a way to learn crafting skills or the delicate art of defusing a bomb in a stress-free environment.

- **Cognitive Skills Targeted by VR Exercises:**
  - **Memory:** Complex VR environments challenge you to recall paths or interpret clues, as if you're a detective piecing together a case based on past events and subtle hints.
  - **Attention:** VR can craft scenarios where distractions abound, demanding concentration akin to a chef keeping track of multiple dishes in a bustling kitchen.
  - **Problem-Solving:** Interactive games equip you with various tools and obstacles, testing your reasoning and adaptability like a chess player strategizing several moves ahead.

- **Feedback and Adaptation Mechanisms in VR:**
    - **Immediate:** The VR world reacts in real-time, providing feedback with each action. It's like a dance where the music changes with your steps, teaching you to move with grace and precision.
    - **Long-Term:** Your progress is tracked and analyzed, allowing the virtual scenarios to evolve with you as a skateboarder's ramps are adjusted with their growing skill.

In this way, VR technology doesn't just engage—it transforms practice into tangible improvements in mental agility, creating a customizable mental gymnasium that is as fun as it is beneficial. Through this dynamic interplay, users can see mental growth and enjoy the journey of development, making the abstract concept of cognitive enhancement a hands-on, immersive experience.

Research in virtual environments, particularly those like Dr. Adam Gazzaley's custom-designed video games, illustrates a practical avenue for cognitive enhancement via neuroplasticity. These games are not meant for entertainment alone; they're developed based on neuroscience principles to specifically target and strengthen cognitive skills. By engaging players in tasks that adapt in real-time to their performance, the games provide a form of mental conditioning that goes beyond play.

For instance, a game may require the player to multitask under changing levels of complexity, which could potentially help improve their working memory and attention span. The underlying technology adjusts the game's difficulty based on real-time performance, ensuring that the player is consistently challenged—never too easy to cause boredom, nor too hard to induce frustration.

The effectiveness of these cognitive training games hinges on their capacity to induce neuroplastic changes. When a player focuses on a task and receives immediate feedback, their brain's neural networks are being exercised and reconfigured. This can lead to improvements in cognitive functions that are not only measurable within the game environment but also transferable to everyday life activities.

While the potential of these virtual environments is significant, it's important to note that they are an evolving technology. Research is ongoing to understand the full scope of benefits and any limitations. Dr. Gazzaley's work, however, already provides promising evidence that such games can be a powerful tool in enhancing mental agility through deliberate practice and brain training.

Let's zoom in on the cognitive landscape shaped by Dr. Adam Gazzaley's video games and explore their foundations in neuroplasticity. These games are like targeted workouts for your brain, each designed with specific mental muscles in mind. They go beyond simple memory or puzzle games; they are constructed on solid neuroscience principles to specifically challenge and develop defined cognitive domains.

- **Attention:** Imagine a game where you're a traffic controller at a busy intersection. The game tasks mimic situations that require vigilant focus, directing the brain to filter out distractions—much like keeping a keen eye out for jaywalkers while managing multiple stoplights.

- **Working Memory:** Picture a scenario where you're a chef remembering orders and cooking meals simultaneously. Such a game improves the brain's 'mental notepad,' enhancing the ability to juggle and update multiple pieces of information.

- **Goal Management:** Consider a complex strategy game that demands constant adjustment of tactics. This is akin to planning a road trip with multiple destinations, promoting the brain's ability to strategize, prioritize, and execute plans efficiently.

The neural circuits engaged by these exercises are not random; they are selected through evidence-based research that identifies which brain networks support different cognitive functions. Like a maestro leading an orchestra, the game's feedback mechanisms guide the neural symphony to either heighten or soften the activity, leading to strengthened connectivity and refined performance over time.

Feedback within these games is as immediate as the echo of a shout in a canyon, allowing players to adjust their strategy in real time. This real-time feedback takes on various forms—points, levels, or visual and auditory cues that signal success or the need for a change in approach.

Through repetitive play, these circuits begin to reshape and improve through a process known as experience-dependent neuroplasticity, much like a path in a forest becomes more defined with frequent travel. Measurable outcomes, such as increased speed in decision-making or a higher accuracy in task performance, signal enhancement in the targeted cognitive domain. It's this bridge between the virtual challenges and real-world cognitive improvement that marks the success of neuroplasticity-based game designs.

By revealing the intricate dance between task, feedback, brain activity, and ensuing neuroplasticity, we can appreciate both the promises and current limitations of these games as tools for cognitive training. While the technology continues to evolve, the progress made thus far offers an enlightening glimpse into the untapped potential of our own brains when paired with the right digital environment.

Brain-computer interfaces (BCIs), neurofeedback, and virtual exercises play increasingly vital roles in medical and educational fields by leveraging the brain's capacity to change, known as neuroplasticity. BCIs help rehabilitate post-injury patients by allowing them to operate prosthetic limbs or computer cursors through neural signals, effectively bypassing damaged physical pathways. This not only aids in regaining lost functionality but also reinforces new neural connections that compensate for the injury.

Neurofeedback serves as a real-time training system that enables individuals with developmental disorders, such as ADHD, to gain greater control over their cognitive functions. By receiving immediate feedback on their brain waves, patients learn to modulate their brain activity, often leading to improvements in focus and a decrease in hyperactivity.

In classroom settings, virtual exercises present an immersive learning environment. Such exercises can transform abstract concepts into interactive experiences, thereby enhancing students' engagement and retention. For instance, a history lesson can come alive in a virtual reality simulation, allowing students to witness historical events firsthand, which can deepen understanding and memory retention.

These modern tools have a common thread in that they convert abstract neural processes into tangible experiences or actions. The success of these technologies in fostering real-world skills underscores the brain's remarkable adaptability and opens up avenues for further applications that can revolutionize rehabilitation, therapy, and learning.

Brain-computer interfaces (BCIs), neurofeedback, and virtual reality (VR) exercises each tap into the brain's neuroplasticity, its inherent ability to reorganize and form new neural connections throughout life.

Starting with BCIs, they often use motor signals from the user's brain to control prosthetic limbs. These neural signals, typically originating in the motor cortex, are detected by electrodes and translated into movements. It's similar to how your hand instinctively grasps a falling cup. The repeated use of BCIs can reinforce new pathways in the brain's motor areas, compensating for the damaged ones, and results can be measured in improved motor function in patients.

Next, neurofeedback for managing ADHD focuses on brain wave modulation. The process uses EEG to monitor the brain's electrical activity and teaches patients to increase or decrease specific brain waves associated with concentration, like the beta waves. It's akin to tuning an instrument to produce the desired sound. This adjustment of brain activity aims to improve focus and reduce impulsivity, akin to practicing quieting the mind amidst noise. Researchers have observed changes in brain wave patterns and improvements in attention tasks, indicating the brain's adaptation.

Lastly, VR in educational settings provides multisensory experiences that engage multiple brain areas, like visual and auditory cortices, to enhance learning. Imagine a history student not just reading about ancient Rome but walking its streets in VR. The sensory immersion and interactive elements of VR can improve knowledge retention and motivation, as seen in studies comparing VR learning outcomes to traditional methods.

Through targeted exercises in these high-tech environments, the brain learns new ways of operating, much like muscles strengthen with exercise. BCIs, neurofeedback, and VR exercises don't just apply to tasks at hand; they can induce lasting changes, strengthening cognitive functions and potentially counteracting impairments. Examples include stroke survivors regaining mobility faster with BCI therapy, and ADHD patients reducing symptoms through neurofeedback training. As research progresses, the evidence supporting these claims continues to grow, solidifying the role of technology-assisted neuroplasticity in rehabilitation and education.

When it comes to technologies that interface with the human brain, a range of ethical considerations naturally arise. Issues of privacy are at the forefront; there's the valid concern about how personal neural data is handled. If we liken neural information to emails in an inbox, it's easy to understand why unauthorized access or misuse could be invasive.

Autonomy is another area under scrutiny. As BCI technologies progress, the question becomes: how much control over their own thoughts and actions do individuals retain when connected to a machine? It's essential to maintain a clear 'user agreement' on who holds the steering wheel in this partnership between human and technology.

The dynamics of human-machine integration further complicate ethics. There's a delicate balance between using these tools to empower people, such as restoring mobility or enhancing cognitive abilities, and creating dependencies that could diminish a person's innate capabilities. Here, it's like weighing the benefits of a calculator for complex math against the potential loss of arithmetic skills through overreliance.

As with any frontier technology, a responsible approach involves openly addressing these ethical challenges, setting up rigorous standards for data protection, informed consent, and ensuring that human-machine cooperation remains just that—a cooperation with human well-being at its core. It's about advancing our capabilities without compromising the values that make us human.

Let's take a deeper look at the intricate web of strategies being woven to safeguard our neural privacy as brain-computer interface (BCM) technologies evolve. Consider your brain's electrical signals as the most personal conversations you have, with BCI technologies akin to a telephone that can dial into those discussions. To protect these, encryption is becoming a standard, turning your neural data into a code that's as indecipherable as a mystery language without the key. Similarly, strict access controls are being developed, similar to having a secure lock on a diary, preventing unauthorized reading of your neural 'pages.'

On the front of autonomy, imagine a scenario where a BCI user is the captain of a ship, with the technology serving as a first mate. Guidelines being developed emphasize that it's the captain who makes the calls, ensuring the technology assists but does not override. This approach preserves the person's decision-making power, keeping them firmly in charge of their cognitive ship.

Considerable discourse is happening around the societal fabric shaped by the integration of BCIs. Much like how overusing a GPS may dull our natural sense of direction, there's concern that certain skills may weaken through dependency on BCIs. Ethicists, policymakers, and technologists are engaged in robust discussions, setting boundaries to harvest the benefits without losing the essence of human ability.

This ongoing conversation seeks to draw lines that are adaptive, just as city zoning evolves with its population's needs. The goal is to maintain a symbiotic relationship between human cognitive strengths and machine-provided opportunities without tipping the balance too far in either direction.

Understanding this nuanced topic means recognizing both the power and the vulnerability inherent in merging our minds with machines. By threading the needle carefully, we can stitch a future that respects individuality, privacy, and personal growth even as we embrace technological assistance. And in doing so, we uphold the human qualities that connect us all, ensuring that these astonishing advances empower rather than inhibit what it means to be human.

As this chapter closes, we stand on the brink of a new era, where the fusion of neuroplasticity and advanced technology holds transformative potential. Think of the brain's ability to rewire itself, and now amplify that with technologies that can guide, enhance, and accelerate this process. The future possibilities are vast.

This synergetic relationship might redefine our approaches to learning, allowing educational systems to tailor experiences that adapt to individual neural patterns, optimizing the way knowledge is acquired and retained. In healthcare, integrating technology with the brain's healing mechanisms could lead to unprecedented recovery methods for neurological injuries, providing customized rehabilitation that evolves with a patient's progress.

And as for personal growth, imagine self-improvement not just as a philosophical pursuit but as a tangible journey, where advancing technology equips us with the means to sculpt our cognitive abilities, emotional resilience, and overall mental fitness. These developments challenge us to reimagine the boundaries of human potential and consider how we might evolve in tandem with the tools we create.

COGNITIVE AND EMOTIONAL ASPECTS

Taking a look at the cognitive and emotional aspects of Neuroplasticity is important. Cognitive efforts, like solving puzzles, and emotional experiences, like the joy of success or frustration of failure, both shape and are shaped by these neural pathways. What we understand now about neuroplasticity not only charts a course for innovative therapies to heal and educate but also highlights the incredible, lifelong capacity of our brains to evolve.

Synaptic strengthening, or long-term potentiation, involves the enhancement of communication between neurons. When we learn something new, such as solving a complex puzzle, the synapses – or contact points for sending signals – become more efficient at transmitting information.

Neurogenesis adds another layer to neuroplasticity. It is the formation of new neurons, particularly in the hippocampus, an area of the brain associated with memory and learning. Engaging in challenging cognitive tasks and enriching environments can stimulate the production of these new neurons, which then integrate into existing neural circuits.

Emotional experiences also play a crucial role in shaping the brain's architecture. Facing and overcoming adversity, for example, can lead to the release of neurotrophins, proteins that support neuron survival and synaptic plasticity. This process fortifies the brain's resilience to future stressors.

Throughout life's stages, from infancy through old age, these neuroplastic changes facilitate learning and adaptation. In childhood, the brain's plasticity helps in acquiring language and social skills; in adulthood, it allows for the continuous learning necessary to navigate an ever-changing environment.

Our expanding knowledge of neuroplasticity is informing new therapeutic approaches for neurological disorders. For individuals who have suffered a stroke, for instance, targeted rehabilitation exercises can help reclaim lost functions by encouraging the formation of new neural connections around the damaged area.

In sum, the brain's remarkable ability to reorganize itself is a testament to its dynamic and responsive nature, empowering us to learn, heal, and grow throughout our lives. Understanding these processes offers hope for innovative treatments that can tap into our brain's innate potential for change.

Just like a master chef combines a variety of spices and ingredients to perfect a dish, each of our emotions and thoughts adds a distinctive flavor to the brain's functioning. Joy might sprinkle sweetness into our day, like a dash of sugar, while anxiety could be the bitter herb that prompts caution. Cognitive tasks, such as working through a challenging problem, mix in complexity much like a robust spice blend. Over time, as we experience and learn new things, our brain incorporates these flavors into its repertoire, fine-tuning the recipe of our mind's operations. It's a continuous process of adaptation, where the mind, much like a kitchen, becomes a place of creativity and exploration, shaped by every thought and emotion we pour into it.

Looking deeper at the complex dance of chemicals in our brain that choreograph our emotional highs and lows, and our cognitive peaks and valleys. When we encounter a moment of joy, it's like hitting the jackpot on a slot machine, and our brain rewards us by releasing dopamine, a feel-good neurotransmitter. This dopamine surge is a pat on the back, encouraging us to seek out similar positive experiences in the future.

Now, consider stress - it's the alarm bell that sounds off in our body, releasing cortisol. Like a city preparing for a storm, cortisol puts us on high alert, heightening our senses and readiness. While this is helpful in short bursts, constant stress can be like a flood, overwhelming the city's defenses and potentially leading to issues like anxiety or depression.

As for the brain's adaptability, think of it as a network of pathways in a vast forest. Each thought or emotion is a traveler, treading along these paths. Frequent travelers along the same route trample the undergrowth, creating a well-worn path that's easier to travel in the future. This is similar to how frequently repeated thoughts or responses can reinforce neural pathways, making them the default routes for our mental processes.

When it comes to learning or healing from trauma, our brain is a resilient gardener that can cultivate new paths or repair damaged ones. If an old path is blocked due to injury, it can redirect travelers to new or less-used paths, training these routes until they become just as easy to traverse. This reflects how our brain adapts to new circumstances, continually reshaping its own landscape to function optimally.

Understanding these neurochemical processes and their influence on our cognition and emotions is like having a map of that forest. It allows us to navigate the terrain wisely, seeking paths that lead to growth and learning while avoiding those that may cause us harm. It's a powerful reminder that with each thought and feeling, we have the opportunity to forge new paths and shape the journey ahead.

Temple Grandin, renowned for her unique cognitive abilities that stem from her autism, provides an exceptional case study in blending perception and emotion to drive change. Grandin's gift for visual thought allowed her to empathize deeply with animals, leading to groundbreaking improvements in livestock handling systems, designed to reduce stress and fear. Her work exemplifies how combining different ways of thinking with emotional insight can result in innovative solutions to complex problems.

This synergy of cognition and emotion is not limited to animal welfare; it extends to various sectors where empathy can inform design, such CREATE as user experience in technology or patient care in healthcare. Grandin's example encourages us to consider diverse perspectives and the emotional context of those we aim to serve, fostering inclusive practices that benefit both the individual and society at large. Her influence shows that harnessing cognitive and emotional synergy has boundless potential, urging us to tap into our unique human capacities in the pursuit of progress and understanding.

Here is the breakdown of Temple Grandin's unique approach that merges cognitive expertise with emotional empathy to revolutionize animal welfare, and its repercussions beyond:

- **Temple Grandin's Cognitive-Emotional Approach to Animal Welfare:**
    - **Visual Thinking:**

- Grandin's mind paints vivid pictures, enabling her to see the world through an animal's eyes. Just like someone might navigate a maze using a map, she uses her spatial awareness to design environments conducive to animal well-being.
  - **Design Features in Livestock Systems:**
  - **Curved Chutes:**
    - Modeled like the arms of a comforting hug, these guide animals naturally, reducing fear.
  - **Non-Slip Flooring:**
    - As safety grips keep a person steady on a slick surface, so does texture on floors stop animals from panicking.
  - **Solid Side Walls:**
    - Mirroring sunglasses that block out distractions, these walls keep animals focused and calm.

- **Emotional States Targeted by These Features:**
  - **Stress Reduction:**
    - Much like a serene landscape soothes the soul, these features maintain a peaceful atmosphere for the animals.
  - **Fear Alleviation:**
    - Providing assurance as a nightlight does to a scared child, the designs aim to minimize the animals' fear.

- **Applications in Other Sectors:**
  - **User Experience Design in Technology:**
    - Grandin's principles teach us that by understanding the users' perspectives – their 'emotional landscape' – designers can create intuitive, user-friendly interfaces.
  - **Patient Care in Healthcare:**
    - Like a gentle bedside manner improves patient comfort, her approach encourages healthcare environments that are empathetic and conducive to healing.

- **Broader Social and Ethical Implications:**
  - **Improved Welfare Standards:**
    - These practices serve as a guide, much like a blueprint for societal compassion, raising standards across industries.
  - **Emotional Intelligence in Design:**
    - Grandin's work illuminates the potential when the tools of empathy are wielded skillfully, crafting solutions that respect both mind and heart.

Through this lens, Grandin's work demonstrates not only a blueprint for animal welfare but also an ethos for human advancement, where understanding and compassion are as critical to design as any material. It's a philosophy that sees every individual – be they human or animal – as part of a larger, interwoven tapestry of experience, deserving of consideration and care.

Mastering a new language or bouncing back from a sports injury are both feats of the brain's adaptability, showcasing neuroplasticity at work. Imagine the brain as a living, flexible puzzle that can rearrange its pieces to face new challenges. When learning a language, each new word or grammar rule is like finding a puzzle piece in a scavenger hunt; with repetition and practice, these pieces click into place, gradually forming a complete picture. Emotions like the satisfaction of stringing together a fluent sentence, or frustration with tricky pronunciation, serve as the fuel that drives this cognitive endeavor, forging stronger connections within the brain.

Similarly, recovering from an injury involves re-mapping the brain's physical coordination and movements. It's like rerouting traffic in a busy city after a main road closes; alternative pathways emerge to keep cars moving. This process requires not only physical therapy but emotional grit—perseverance despite pain and the belief in regaining strength. The brain takes cues from these emotional and cognitive strategies, rewiring and enhancing connections to muscles and nerves, thereby facilitating healing.

Whether it's language acquisition or healing, both journeys are underpinned by the intertwining of thought processes and emotional stamina, the twin engines driving the incredible neural changes that define neuroplasticity. It is a testament to our capacity for transformation, powered by the intricate interplay of our minds and hearts.

Let's take a deeper look at the orchestra of the brain's activity when learning a new language and healing from an injury. In the realm of language acquisition, the brain's Broca's and Wernicke's areas are the conductors of our linguistic symphony, orchestrating the production and comprehension of new words and phrases. Imagine these brain regions lighting up like a concert hall's stage as they actively engage in the language-learning process. Mastering a language spotlights these areas, increasing their synaptic connections, like adding more musicians to the stage to enrich the performance.

When it comes to recovering from a sports injury, the brain is a seasoned coach, guiding the rehabilitation of motor skills. The motor cortex, responsible for voluntary movement, adapts through a process similar to a team developing new gameplay strategies. It forms new connections and bolsters existing ones in response to physical therapy, akin to a quarterback throwing passes to new receivers. Neurotrophic factors, which are like the brain's personal training staff, support neural regeneration and synaptic plasticity, ensuring the injured region is encouraged to strengthen and heal.

Emotional resilience in this context is akin to the crowd's support during a comeback game. It fuels the brain's motivation and persistence, cheering on the neurons as they forge new pathways or re-establish old ones, reinforcing the brain's capacity to overcome and adapt. This combination of cognitive strategies, supported by emotional fortitude, allows us to not only recover but also to emerge with new skills and strengths, showcasing the limitless potential of the human brain when it comes to learning and healing.

Consider the possibilities as advances in neuroplasticity—understanding how our brains change through cognitive and emotional experiences—reshape our methods in education, personal development, and injury recovery. This knowledge equips us with the tools to create educational programs that are tailored to how the brain actually learns, fostering environments where mental agility and emotional intelligence are nurtured. For personal growth, the implications are profound: we can develop strategies that capitalize on our brain's natural plasticity to foster resilience and adaptability. In terms of healing, the insights from neuroplasticity can revolutionize rehabilitation, making the journey from injury to recovery more efficient and effective. Embracing these insights promises to unlock human potential in ways we are only beginning to imagine.

In wrapping up this chapter, we reflect on the dynamic interplay between cognitive processes and emotional states, and how this synergy contributes to the brain's remarkable ability to adapt and evolve. By understanding this relationship, we are better positioned to harness the potential of our own minds, tailoring educational approaches, personal development techniques, and recovery protocols that align with our innate neuroplastic capabilities. This knowledge empowers us not only to overcome challenges but also to thrive, enriching our lives with continued learning and growth. Through embracing the principles of neuroplasticity, we open doors to a future where our cognitive and emotional faculties are more integrated and effectively utilized, enabling us to lead lives that are fuller, more resilient, and deeply interconnected.

THE AGING BRAIN AND PLASTICITY

The brain, even as we age, is not a static organ bound to decline; it is dynamic and capable of continuous adaptation and learning. This ability, known as neuroplasticity, was once thought to be the domain of the young. Yet, current understanding affirms that our neural networks can be refined and reshaped throughout our lives. This negates the outdated belief that older adults are unable to learn as effectively as their younger counterparts. The aging brain maintains the primary function of adapting to new knowledge and environments, ensuring that learning and cognitive development are lifelong processes. Acknowledging this capacity is crucial for promoting strategies that support brain health in older adults and redefining societal norms about aging and cognition.

Synaptic plasticity, which includes both long-term potentiation (LTP) and long-term depression (LTD), refers to the strengthening or weakening of synapses, the junctions between neurons where communication occurs. Think of LTP as reinforcing a bridge so that traffic flows more easily, a process essential for learning and memory. Conversely, LTD is like reducing traffic over a bridge that's less frequently used, a crucial process for forgetting and unlearning.

Neurotrophic factors such as BDNF are the construction workers of the brain's plasticity. BDNF, for instance, supports the survival of neurons, encouraging the growth of new synapses and strengthening existing ones. It's somewhat like a fertilizer that promotes growth and health in a garden.

Dendritic branching and synaptogenesis involve the growth of new dendrites, the tree branch-like extensions of neurons, and the formation of new synaptic connections. This process is akin to expanding the roots and branches of a tree to reach new sources of sunlight and nutrients, enhancing the tree's (or brain's) capacity to thrive.

Various stimuli, including physical exercise, mental challenges, and social interactions, can enhance or deter these neuroplastic processes—similar to how a plant's growth is influenced by light exposure, water, and soil quality.

In practice, cognitive behavioral therapy (CBT) makes use of neuroplasticity by helping individuals reframe their thoughts, effectively rewiring patterns of thinking to alleviate mental distress. Skill acquisition practices, from playing an instrument to juggling, rely on the brain's plasticity to solidify the neural pathways necessary for these complex tasks.

By understanding these mechanisms, we can appreciate how the brain maintains and improves cognitive health over time, adapting continuously to the complexities of our environment and experiences.

The common belief that aging inevitably leads to a steep decline in cognitive abilities is being refuted by new evidence that highlights the brain's enduring capacity to learn and change, even in later years. Recent studies have shown that the creation of new neurons, known as neurogenesis, and the brain's ability to restructure itself, a process called neuroplasticity, persist well into older age. It's akin to the body's ability to heal a wound at any age: the process might slow down a bit, but it doesn't stop. These findings debunk the myth that seniors are bound to cognitive deterioration and instead paint a more accurate picture of an adaptable brain that continues to forge new connections and pathways. This scientific understanding reinforces the value of lifelong learning and the potential for continued intellectual growth, suggesting that with the right stimulation and activities, the senior brain can remain both active and resilient.

Let's take a deeper dive into the fascinating landscape of the aging brain, where the rigors of time don't mean an end to learning and growth. Picture the brain not as an old machine set in its ways but more like a seasoned artist, continually creating new strokes on the canvas of neural pathways. Even as we age, our brain is bustling like a city under constant renovation—building new bridges (synapses) that connect different neighborhoods (neural networks).

The city's construction materials come in the form of neurotrophic factors, such as BDNF, which is like a supercharged nutrient that helps strengthen and build new structures (neurons and synapses). And just like a city, the brain thrives on activity; learning a new language or musical instrument lays down fresh neural pavement, ensuring the traffic of thoughts and memories flows more smoothly.

These activities are akin to the workout a top athlete undertakes, except the gym is the mind, and the exercise is cognitive engagement. Consistent mental activity sharpens the brain's capabilities, keeping the cognitive cogs well-oiled and efficient. It is in these seemingly simple acts of engagement—like mastering the latest smartphone or joining a book club—where we see the profound effect on the brain's structure and function, a testament to its adaptable nature.

This understanding isn't just academic; it has real-world implications. We see it applied in strategies like cognitive behavioral therapy, which subtly reshapes thought patterns, or in rehabilitation programs that help older adults regain functions lost to injury. These practical applications root themselves in the truth that our brains, no matter the age, are dynamic and malleable, capable of transformation and resilience.

Embracing this can shift how we view aging, seeing it not as a winding down but as an opportunity for continued development, where each new challenge is a chance to reinforce and expand the neural networks that shape who we are. It's a message that injects vibrancy into the prospect of growing older, knowing that our mental faculties can flourish well into our twilight years.

Continuing to learn and participate in activities that challenge the mind is vital for sustaining brain health as we age. Much like a muscle that strengthens with exercise, the brain benefits from engagement in tasks that stimulate thought and require mental effort. Engaging in puzzles, learning new skills, or even reading regularly can activate various brain areas, keeping them in good working order. These activities are not trivial; they contribute to the creation of new neural pathways and the strengthening of existing ones, which is essential for cognitive agility.

Evidence suggests that such sustained cognitive engagement can have a protective effect against the decline in cognitive abilities often associated with aging. It can help maintain memory, problem-solving skills, and even improve the speed of processing information. In practice, this could translate to a more independent life, with a reduced risk of developing neurocognitive disorders.

Moreover, these cognitive exercises may contribute positively to emotional well-being. For example, mastering a new hobby can provide a sense of accomplishment and confidence, making it not just a tool for maintaining cognitive functions, but also for enhancing the quality of life. This proactive approach to brain health advocates for a lifestyle that integrates continuous learning and mental challenges as cornerstones for healthy aging.

Let's take a deeper look at the intricacies of the aging brain's ability to reshape itself through learning and cognitive exercise. Imagine each new task or bit of information as a spark in the neural network, similar to striking a match to illuminate a dark room. In the senior brain, these sparks of activity help forge new pathways and reinforce existing ones, ensuring the lights keep burning bright.

As older adults engage in cognitive exercises, their brains undergo a renovative process. Take memory-enhancing activities, for instance—these are like mental push-ups that strengthen the hippocampus, the brain's memory storage room. Or consider problem-solving tasks that speed up information transmission along neural pathways, much like upgrading the wiring in an old house to restore and improve its electricity flow.

During these activities, the brain releases a cocktail of neurochemicals. One of them, dopamine, acts like a reward system booster, encouraging the continuation of the learning process. Another, BDNF, serves as brain fertilizer, supporting the growth and maintenance of neural connections.

This change is not limited to the microscopic level. It's reflected in broader shifts in brain activity patterns, which can be seen on neuroimaging scans. These scans reveal the before and after effects of consistent cognitive training, like comparing satellite images of a city before and after implementing a new public park system.

By maintaining a regimen of learning and mental challenges, seniors can not only protect against cognitive decline but also enhance their brain capabilities. Just as an experienced gardener knows which seeds to sow for a bountiful harvest, so too can individuals learn which activities will best nourish their neural landscapes for lasting brain health and emotional well-being.

The brain's ability to forge new paths and connections can be likened to a vibrant, ever-growing tree, branching out in new directions. For the elderly, each cognitive exercise is akin to the natural growth of a tree's branches reaching for sunlight. Just as the limbs and leaves stretch upwards and outwards, finding new spaces to flourish, the brain, too, reaches out with neural extensions, seeking new connections and experiences.

Similarly, consistent cognitive exercises for the elderly are comparable to a regular regimen of strength training for the body. Engaging in puzzles, learning new languages, or even daily reading acts as a weightlifting session for the brain, fortifying neural circuits the way muscles strengthen with use. Over time, just as muscles become more robust and versatile, the tasks that once seemed challenging become easier for the brain to manage, demonstrating the plasticity and resilience of our cognitive 'musculature'.

This growth and strengthening of neural connections are essential for maintaining brain health, helping to keep cognitive decline at bay, much like how physical exercise preserves the body's vitality. Each new learning experience for an older adult is not just a moment of personal achievement, but a tangible expansion of their mental acuity, showcasing how the brain, regardless of age, remains capable of remarkable feats of adaptation and development.

Here's a detailed breakdown of the cognitive rejuvenation that comes from engaging the aging brain in mental gymnastics:

- **Cognitive Processes Influenced:**
    - Memory enhancement: Like sharpening an old pencil to write a new chapter, mental exercises can help the mind record and recall with better clarity.
    - Problem-solving skills: Training the brain with puzzles is akin to a detective honing their investigation skills, ensuring mental agility.
    - Information processing: Quick-witted banter isn't just for the young; like upgrading an old computer, mental activities can speed up cognitive processing.

- **Stimulated Neural Pathways:**
    - Sensory pathways: Engaging with complex textures or sounds can upgrade the brain's sensory highway, much like adding lanes to a road.

- Motor skills pathways: Fine motor activities such as crafts or writing call to mind the intricate dance between thought and action, refining the brain's control center.

- Emotional processing pathways: Understanding and expressing emotions can be compared to painting with a diverse palette, enriching the brain's emotional landscape.

- **Increasing Synaptic Strength:**
- Activity-dependent synaptic plasticity: Regular brain activities act as a workout routine for neural connections, enhancing their strength and efficiency.

- **Roles of Brain Regions:**
- Hippocampus: Just as a librarian organizes books, this region helps store and retrieve memories.
- Prefrontal cortex: For strategizing and planning, this area is like a seasoned chess player considering their next move.
- Amygdala: In processing emotions, it acts like the heart of the brain's emotional responses.

- **Overall Impact on Cognitive Health:**
- Enhanced mental resilience: Continuous learning builds a robust mental framework, similar to constructing a sturdier house that withstands storms.
- Reduced risk of neurodegenerative diseases: Keeping the mind active is like fortifying city walls, offering protection against potential invaders.

- **Reinforcement Through Repetition:**
- Just as practicing a song on a guitar makes the fingers remember the chords, repetition in mental tasks ingrains the neural patterns, making recall second nature.

- **Supporting Neurochemicals:**
- BDNF: This neurotrophic factor nurtures the brain's neurons and connections like water and sunlight to plants.
- Dopamine: The feel-good neurotransmitter that rewards learning and discovery, much like the satisfaction of solving a riddle.

- **Long-term Benefits:**
- Cognitive function: Continuous mental challenge keeps the brain youthful, like regular tune-ups keep a classic car cruising smoothly.
- Emotional well-being: The pride in mastering new skills buoys the

spirits, akin to the joy from cultivating a thriving garden.

By engaging in this array of cognitive exercises, older adults can effectively remodel the mental blueprint of their brains, promoting a landscape of thought that is fertile and flourishing even in the golden years.

Activities and habits that foster neuroplasticity are essential for maintaining cognitive health, functioning akin to proactive maintenance for complex machinery. Good nutrition, for instance, provides the brain with essential nutrients, acting as high-quality fuel that enables it to perform optimally. Regular exercise increases blood flow to the brain, which can be compared to improving the transportation network of a bustling city, allowing for better delivery of nutrients and removal of waste. Additionally, mental exercises through lifelong learning constantly challenge the brain, similar to how regular software updates add new features and improve performance on a computer.

These practices contribute to the brain's ability to adapt and grow by enhancing neural connections and promoting the formation of new ones. Engaging in such activities can sharpen memory, improve attention, and increase mental fluidity. The benefits extend beyond preserving cognitive function; they also include a reduction in the risk of cognitive decline and an overall positive impact on mental wellbeing.

Consistently integrating these nourishing activities and habits into one's lifestyle is not merely about preventing deterioration; it's about investing in the longevity and vitality of one's mental capabilities, much like regularly servicing a car to ensure it runs well for years to come. As new research continues to shed light on neuroplasticity, incorporating these foundational practices becomes even more pivotal for a healthy, active brain throughout all stages of life.

Let's take a deeper look at the remarkable transformations our brains undergo with lifestyle choices that promote neuroplasticity. Imagine your brain as a garden; consuming a diet rich in omega-3 fatty acids is like using premium soil that keeps the plants—the neurons—healthy and robust. Antioxidants work similarly to a protective shield, guarding the plants from damaging elements, which in the brain's case helps prevent neuronal damage and supports the creation of new synapses, like budding flowers in the spring.

Aerobic exercise, on the other hand, can be compared to a revitalizing rain shower that not only waters the garden but also enriches it with vital nutrients. It boosts neurogenesis, encouraging the growth of new neuronal seedlings. This physical activity also elevates levels of BDNF, which is like a growth serum that helps these new neurons and synapses flourish.

Now, consider the brain engagement that comes from cognitive tasks such as strategic games or learning new skills. It's akin to a series of challenges that prompt the garden's plants to extend their roots and branches, intertwining and becoming more complex and resilient, creating a luscious, interconnected network.

These activities are more than just daily routines; they're investments in the brain's health and capability to recover from injuries, like a well-attended garden that bounces back quicker from harsh weather. Engaging regularly in mentally stimulating activities ensures that the brain's intricate network of synaptic connections remains active and pliable, ready to repair and strengthen as needed, ensuring that cognitive functions are not merely maintained but can also be reclaimed after damage or decline. Through these insights, we appreciate the profound impact of our actions on our brain's health and the ever-unfolding potential that our neural landscape holds.

Older adults around the world are shattering the mold of what it means to age, demonstrating the brain's impressive capacity to not just endure, but thrive with new skills and challenges. Take Yuichiro Miura, for example, who, at the age of 80, defied age-related stereotypes by scaling the summit of Mount Everest. His undertaking shows that the brain, like an experienced climber, can still conquer new peaks, mastering the skills needed to navigate unprecedented terrain.

Similarly, many seniors today are embracing the world of technology, which, a mere decade ago, might have seemed as alien as a distant galaxy. Their ability to navigate smartphones, social media, and the digital world is like adapting to a new language, transforming the tapestry of their daily lives. These stories serve as vibrant testaments to the brain's elasticity and potential for growth, illustrating how, with determination and the right challenges, the twilight years can become a time of intellectual and personal renaissance. Whether climbing literal mountains or surfing the digital wave, these experiences underline the transformative power of new learning, underscoring that the brain, at any age, is a boundlessly adaptive organ.

Here is the breakdown on the remarkable neuroplastic changes seen in older adults:

- **Types of Neural Adaptations:**
  - Synaptic Plasticity:
    - Increased synaptic strength, like reinforcing a muscle with regular use.
    - Greater synaptic efficacy, akin to improving signal quality in a phone conversation.
  - Growth of New Synapses:
    - Formation of new synaptic connections, similar to building new bridges to previously disconnected islands.
  - Neurogenesis:
    - Creation of new neurons in the brain, as a garden generates new blossoms.
  - Enhanced Neurotrophic Factors:
    - Increase in brain-derived neurotrophic factors (BDNF), much like a boost in vital nutrients for a plant's growth.

- **Structural Changes:**
  - Dendritic Growth:
    - Dendrites, the branches of neurons, expand and grow, akin to the tree's branches spreading to capture more sunlight.
  - Changes in White Matter:
    - Increase in white matter integrity, comparable to upgrading the insulation on electrical cables for better functionality.

- **Functional Changes:**
  - Increased Brain Region Connectivity:
    - Enhanced communication between different brain areas, imagine the upgrade from a dial-up to high-speed internet.
  - Functional Reorganization:
    - Brain areas adapting new roles, like a multifunctional tool evolving with added features.

- **Manifestations Across Cognitive Domains:**
  - Memory:
    - Improved recall and storage, echoing the expansion of a librarian's

catalog system.
  - Spatial Navigation:
    - Better navigational skills, similar to an experienced captain sailing through familiar waters.
  - Executive Function:
    - Sharpened problem-solving capabilities, like a seasoned detective piecing together clues.
  - Attention and Focus:
    - Heightened attention span, paralleling a watchmaker's precision and concentration.

Engagement in new and challenging tasks injects the senior brain with a dose of rejuvenation, akin to updating and upgrading an old yet valuable piece of technology. Whether it's Yuichiro Miura climbing Everest or a grandparent mastering the latest smartphone, such experiences are not merely leisure activities; they are fundamental workouts for the brain, leading to impactful changes that support a vibrant, active mental state well into the golden years of life.

Neuroplasticity holds the key to unlocking an aging brain's vast potential, with profound implications for enhancing quality of life. This innate capacity enables the brain to continually adapt, form new connections, and rewire itself in response to learning and experience. Its primary function is to maintain cognitive agility and resilience, supporting the acquisition of new skills and the retention of knowledge. The impact of neuroplasticity extends to improved memory, heightened problem-solving abilities, and broader emotional well-being. Harnessing this capability can lead to a richer, more fulfilling experience in later years, challenging the misconception that aging necessitates cognitive decline. Embracing a lifestyle that promotes neuroplasticity can furnish the aging brain with the tools to thrive, crafting a narrative of growth and adaptability that defies traditional expectations of aging.

FUTURE FRONTIERS IN NEUROPLASTICITY

While the basics of neuroplasticity are broadly understood, there's still much to learn about its complexities and nuances. Future research may reveal more about how we can enhance and direct this plasticity to improve cognitive health, rehabilitate injuries, and possibly prevent various neurological conditions. This exploration into the mechanics of neuroplasticity invites us to appreciate the remarkable adaptability of the human brain and the substantial possibilities for its further application.

Neuroplasticity in learning and memory works as follows:

1. **Stimulus and Response**: When we encounter new information, our brain cells, called neurons, communicate through electrical and chemical signals. Each neuron can connect with thousands of others, forming a vast and dynamic network.

2. **Synaptic Strengthening**: If two neurons consistently participate in this signaling, the synapse (the point of communication between these neurons) strengthens. This is known as 'synaptic strengthening,' and it's akin to carving a deeper path in the ground the more it's walked upon.

3. **Repetition and Reinforcement**: Repeating an action or recalling knowledge requires these synapses to fire again. Over time, repetition makes these connections more durable and efficient, much like using a trail regularly makes it easier to navigate.

4. **Long-Term Potentiation (LTP)**: With persistent use, certain synaptic connections experience LTP, a long-lasting increase in signal strength between two neurons. It's like increasing the bandwidth of a network connection for faster and clearer communication.

In memory consolidation:

1. **Short-Term to Long-Term**: Short-term memories initially involve transient synaptic changes. Through processes like LTP, these changes can become more permanent, making the memory long-lasting.

2. **Neural Networks**: Over time, networks of neurons that represent memories can alter their structure and function, a process facilitated by neuroplasticity. These networks are like intricate circuits that light up when a specific memory is recalled or a practiced skill is performed.

Neuroplasticity also plays a crucial role in the brain's recovery after injury:

1. **Reorganization**: When one area of the brain is damaged, surrounding regions can sometimes take over its functions, a phenomenon known as plastic reorganization.

2. **Formation of New Connections**: The brain can form new neuronal pathways to bypass damaged areas, similar to creating a detour around a blocked road after a landslide.

Various factors influence neuroplasticity:

1. **Age**: Young brains are typically more plastic, but adults can also improve their brain's malleability with the proper stimuli.

2. **Environment**: Stimulating environments with novel experiences can enhance neuroplasticity.

3. **Genetics**: Individual genetic makeup can dictate one's propensity for neuroplastic change.

Scientists measure and observe neuroplasticity through:

1. **Brain Imaging Techniques**: Such as fMRI, which can visualize changes in brain activity.

2. **Electrophysiological Methods**: Including EEG, which records electrical activity in the brain.

In rehabilitation, therapeutic approaches that leverage neuroplastics include:

1. **Physical Therapy**: Engages neuroplasticity to relearn motor skills.

2. **Cognitive Training**: Uses tasks designed to improve functions like attention and memory.

3. **Technological Interventions**: Such as virtual reality, which can simulate real-life scenarios for therapy.

Advancing our understanding of neuroplasticity has the potential to:

1. **Refine Therapies**: Improve current treatments for brain injuries and cognitive decline.

2. **Develop Preventative Strategies**: Help maintain cognitive function in aging populations.

3. **Cure Neurological Conditions**: Lead to cures for diseases previously thought incurable.

By embracing the nuanced role of neuroplasticity, we can pave the way to remarkable advancements in neurological health and personal well-being.

Think of the brain's neuroplasticity like the software on a smartphone. Just as a phone's operating system is updated to improve functionality or add new features, our brains can also rewire and update themselves to learn new information or skills. Every task we perform, from swiping on a screen to installing a new app, is comparable to the mental tasks we undertake; they contribute to forming new neural connections or strengthening the existing ones, much like habitual use of an app makes its launch command almost second nature to us.

Everyday experiences, like navigating a new city or learning to use a new piece of technology, prompt our brain to adapt, laying down neural pathways as quickly as a phone downloads data to support new functions. This neuroplasticity isn't just about gaining more 'apps' or skills; it's about keeping the 'hardware'—our brain—operating smoothly and efficiently even when faced with potential 'system errors,' like brain injuries or neurodegenerative diseases.

By taking a cue from the uninterrupted improvements in smartphone technology, researchers delving into neuroplasticity aim to find ways to keep our cognitive 'devices' not just up-to-date, but also resilient and adaptive, ready to tackle the ever-changing demands of life with each 'software upgrade' derived from new learning and experience.

Let's take a deeper look at the inner workings of neuroplasticity, starting with synaptic plasticity—the brain's way of adjusting the strength of connections between neurons, much like tuning the strings of a guitar for the perfect pitch. When we learn a new skill or task, our brain cells, or neurons, communicate via tiny structures called synapses. Think of these as miniature docks where the cargo of neurotransmitters is shuttled across to transport messages from one neuron to another. The frequent use of a particular neural pathway, much like repeatedly walking a path through a meadow, makes this synaptic 'dock' more robust and the transmission of neurotransmitters more efficient.

During learning and memory consolidation, not only does the rate of neurotransmitter release escalate, but there's also a change in the receptor density on the post-synaptic neuron—the receiving end of the message. Imagine a bustling marketplace, where more stalls (receptors) open up to meet the increasing demand from customers (neurotransmitters). As this marketplace grows, it becomes easier for information to be exchanged and remembered.

Now, consider brain injury. Just as a community comes together to rebuild after a storm, the brain mobilizes its neuroplastic abilities to repair and reroute connections. Neurons will grow new branches, called dendrites, to re-establish communication with their neighbors, akin to rebuilding roads between towns. They might even form entirely new networks, bypassing damaged areas as cleanly as a detour around a construction site.

At the molecular level, this remarkable process is supported by a symphony of signaling pathways. Proteins like BDNF (brain-derived neurotrophic factor) play a key role here, acting as fertilizer promoting the growth of new synaptic connections and dendrites. Think of BDNF as a nurturing rain that stimulates a parched land to sprout new life—aiding the brain's recovery and rejuvenation.

Environmental factors such as mental stimulation, physical exercise, and even our social environment, act like sunlight, soil, and water—each one crucial for the growth and health of our 'neural garden.' Engaging activities, rich relationships, and regular physical movement can boost neuroplasticity, ensuring our brain's landscape remains fertile and vigorous.

In healthcare, optimizing these elements is like equipping gardeners with the best tools and knowledge. Therapeutic interventions, such as targeted cognitive exercises and rehabilitation programs, are designed not just to maintain the garden but to help it flourish, even in the face of injuries or cognitive diseases. By applying our expanding understanding of neuroplasticity to such therapies, we can hope to nurture the brain's resilience, ensuring a lush and resilient cognitive landscape throughout a person's life.

Transcranial Magnetic Stimulation (TMS) and brain-computer interfaces are two technologies harnessing the brain's plastic capabilities. TMS uses magnetic fields to stimulate specific parts of the brain. Imagine using a magnet to activate a dormant machine; similarly, TMS can target inactive or underperforming regions of the brain, prompting them to 'wake up' and reconnect with the rest of the brain network.

On the other hand, brain-computer interfaces (BCIs) create direct communication pathways between the brain and an external device. Think of a BCI as a translator that interprets your brain's electrical activity and converts these signals into commands to control computers or prosthetics, bridging the gap between thought and action without the need for physical movement.

Both technologies are used not only to understand the brain better but also have therapeutic potentials. For instance, TMS has shown promise in treating depression and other neurological conditions, while BCIs could restore mobility and communication in individuals with severe physical disabilities. While these technologies offer great hope, they also come with limitations and challenges, such as accessibility and the need for individual calibration. As research continues, the potential for these tools to improve lives grows, pivoting on our increasing ability to harness the brain's adaptability.

Here's a breakdown of how Transcranial Magnetic Stimulation and brain-computer interfaces engage with the brain's capacity for change:

Transcranial Magnetic Stimulation (TMS):
- **Magnetic Field Generation**: Like a miniature thunderstorm, TMS induces a concentrated electrical current using a coil placed near the scalp, creating a magnetic field that penetrates the skull unimpeded.
- **Coil Types**: Different coil shapes, such as figure-eight or H-coil, target brain regions with varying precision, like adjusting a camera lens to focus on a subject.
- **Targeting Accuracy**: Precision in TMS is akin to using a GPS to pinpoint a location, targeting specific brain areas involved in different functions.
- **Navigation Systems**: Systems like neuronavigation use brain imaging to guide the positioning of the TMS coil much like street maps guide a driver.
- **Affected Neurons**: TMS influences neurons that are close to the brain's surface, stimulating them to fire impulses, comparable to flicking a switch to light a bulb.
- **Neuron Types**: Preferentially stimulates neurons oriented perpendicular to the direction of the electric field.
- **Neurophysiological Responses**: The brain reacts to this external stimulation by increasing or decreasing the excitability of neurons, not unlike turning the volume up or down on a speaker.
- **Synaptic Changes**: Repetitive stimulation can strengthen or weaken synaptic connections, molding the brain's communication pathways as a river shapes its banks.

Brain-Computer Interfaces (BCIs):
- **Neural Signal Detection**: BCIs detect the brain's electrical chatter by picking up signals through sensors, much like satellites capturing transmission signals.
- **Electrode Placement**: Electrodes can be non-invasively placed on the scalp or implanted for more direct and precise signal capture.
- **Signal Interpretation**: Advanced algorithms decode these signals,

translating them into commands, similar to understanding a foreign language through a translator app.

- **Machine Learning**: These algorithms improve over time, learning to differentiate brain patterns like a student becoming proficient in a new language.

- **Output Execution**: The interpreted signals command external devices, which is analogous to using a remote to control a toy car or a drone.

- **Applications**: This control may extend to computer cursors, robotic arms, or even exoskeletons, granting users the power of action and communication.

Aiding Recovery Post-Injury:

- **Motor Functions**: Both TMS and BCIs have the potential to restore movement by reinforcing new neural pathways—like forging new trails through a forest to reach a destination.

- **Plasticity and Rehabilitation**: Promote the brain's plasticity for motor recovery, guiding it through the relearning process as a coach aids an athlete in regaining form.

- **Communication Abilities**: BCIs can help patients with speech impairments by providing alternative communication methods, akin to unlocking new ways for a silent performer to express themselves.

Both TMS and BCIs represent a frontier in the practical application of neuroplasticity, each with a unique mechanism for tapping into the brain's adaptive power—holding the promise of a future where repairing and enhancing brain function becomes as commonplace as daily communication and interaction.

Dr. Norman Doidge's work with neuroplasticity is a beacon of hope, shedding light on the brain's remarkable capability to change and heal. Just as a dedicated gardener can revive a withered plant, Doidge has shown that, with the right techniques, it may be possible to rehabilitate brains that were once considered irreparable. Through his fascinating case studies—akin to transformational makeovers—we witness stroke victims relearning to speak and walk, much like someone relearning a lost craft.

His books, filled with these narratives, function as guides that debunk the myth of the brain's rigidity, much as a myth-buster show reveals the truth behind urban legends. Doidge's work isn't just about presenting marvels; it's about providing a blueprint for harnessing neuroplasticity, comparable to teaching someone not just to fish but to refine and master the art of fishing.

By translating the science of brain adaptation into stories of personal triumph, Dr. Doidge's contributions resonate on a deeply personal level. They remind us that within our own minds lies a frontier as expansive and promising as space—the final frontier—once seemed to a previous generation of dreamers and explorers. His work continues to inspire both those in the medical field and individuals everywhere to view the human brain not as a static, unchangeable entity, but as a dynamic and evolving organ, full of potential for renewal and growth.

Current research in neuroplasticity is reshaping our approach to medical treatment and cognitive enhancement. In the realm of treatment, the growing understanding of the brain's adaptive capabilities is steering us toward therapies that not only aim to repair damage but actively work with the brain's ability to rewire itself. For instance, stroke rehabilitation programs now incorporate exercises specifically designed to retrain unaffected brain areas to take over functions from damaged ones, much like retraining a backup singer to take center stage when the lead vocalist is unable to perform.

In the sphere of cognitive training, we are developing tools and programs based on neuroplasticity principles to sharpen the mind and address cognitive decline. This research could lead to the creation of "mental gyms" where individuals undertake tailored brain exercises, strengthening their minds as one would strengthen muscles at a physical gym, potentially preventing or delaying dementia and other cognitive impairments.

The implications for everyday life are expansive and profound. From enhancing learning in educational settings to offering new treatment avenues for those struggling with mental health issues, the benefits of tapping into the brain's plastic nature promise to touch every aspect of human endeavor. As we progress, the potential to fine-tune these approaches grows, fostering a future where managing brain health becomes an integrated part of daily life, as routine and vital as maintaining a balanced diet or regular physical exercise.

Let's take a deeper look at how therapies and trainings inspired by neuroplasticity work their magic on the brain. Picture your brain as a dynamic city, where the neural pathways are the roads. During stroke recovery, if one of the main highways is damaged, targeted exercises can be like construction projects, building new roads or strengthening smaller pathways so they can handle more traffic and take on the roles of the damaged routes. This remodeling is made possible by the growth of new synapses, akin to paving new paths, and neurogenesis, which is like constructing new buildings to expand the city's capability.

These exercises are not random; they're designed to work just the challenging enough to push the brain's adaptability without overwhelming it, similar to a workout routine that's tailored to increase muscle strength without causing injury. For enhancing memory and attention, specific cognitive tasks might involve complex problem-solving or memory exercises like trying to navigate a maze or recounting detailed stories from memory, which encourage existing neurons to form stronger, more efficient connections.

The evidence for the success of these therapies and exercises comes from clinical and cognitive assessments, which are the tools used to measure any changes in brain activity and behavior. It's much like using traffic sensors and commuter feedback to determine if new roadways are effective. These assessments can show improvements in areas like reaction times, recall abilities, or the ability to multitask.

In education, mental health treatment, and prevention, integrating neuroplasticity-based approaches means better-customized programs that consider each person's unique brain 'layout.' It's a promising shift towards precision medicine and education, targeting the 'cognitive workout' to fit the specific needs of an individual's brain, potentially leading to broad societal benefits, including more effective treatments, enhanced learning environments, and preventative strategies against cognitive decline. This evolving landscape signifies a future where understanding and improving brain function becomes as integral and personalized as physical fitness and nutrition.

Neuroplasticity research is revolutionizing our understanding of the brain's potential to adapt and recover. Its fundamental principle – that the brain can reorganize itself in response to experiences and challenges – is reshaping our approaches to learning, therapy, and self-improvement. We now know that through targeted exercises and interventions, it's possible to forge new neural pathways and enhance brain function, offering hope for recovery from injuries and neurological conditions that were once considered permanent. This evolving field is not only crucial for patients undergoing rehabilitation but also has significant implications for the general population, as we seek to optimize mental agility and cognitive health across the lifespan. The promise of neuroplasticity extends into every corner of human life, indicating that our capacity to grow, evolve, and heal is far greater than previously imagined.

CONCLUSION

As we close the final pages of "Neuroplasticity Made Easy," we can reflect on the journey through the fascinating landscape of the human brain. We've discovered the vast potential of neuroplasticity, learning how our neural pathways can be rewired and strengthened throughout our lives. The key themes of adaptability, growth, and the transformative power of consistent practice have emerged as cornerstones of a mentally resilient life.

The lessons learned here extend beyond mere theory, offering practical applications that can influence how we learn, cope with challenges, and recover from setbacks. By understanding and embracing the principles of neuroplasticity, we've gained valuable insights into improving our cognitive functions, developing healthier habits, and approaching brain health with renewed optimism.

The overarching impact of this book is a message of empowerment. It illuminates the idea that no matter our age or circumstances, there is always room for change and improvement. Our brains are not fixed entities but works in progress, responsive to our actions and attitudes.

As you step back into the world, armed with this knowledge, consider the endless possibilities that lie within your neural connections. The road to cognitive enhancement and better brain health is lifelong and, as you've learned, wholly within your control. Let the insights from "Neoperlasticity Made Easy" be a compass that guides you toward a future where the incredible plasticity of your brain is not just understood but fully harnessed in pursuit of your goals and dreams.

ABOUT THE AUTHOR

Jon Adams brings a wealth of experience from over twenty years in the information technology industry, having worked with some of the world's leading tech giants. With a deep-seated passion for science, technology, and languages, Jon excels at demystifying complex subjects, making them accessible and engaging to a broad audience.

His writings focus on breaking down intricate topics into everyday terms, helping readers not just learn but also apply this knowledge in their daily lives.

Currently, Jon is a proud member of Green Mountain Computing, which publishes his insightful books. Through his work, he aims to foster a deeper understanding and appreciation of technology and science, enriching readers' lives.

Jon@GreenMountainComputing.com

www.ingramcontent.com/pod-product-compliance
Lightning Source LLC
Chambersburg PA
CBHW052333220526
45472CB00001B/400